THE CARNIVORE INSTINCT
COOKBOOK FOR BEGINNERS

Unleash the Power of the Meat-Based Diet with 80 Delectable Recipes for Your Natural Healing, Optimal Health, and Effortless Weight Loss

Garrett Lane

© **Copyright 2024 Garrett Lane – All rights reserved.**

The content contained within this book may not be reproduced, duplicated, or transmitted without direct written permission from the author or the publisher.

Under no circumstances will any blame or legal responsibility be held against the publisher or author for any damages, reparation, or monetary loss due to the information contained within this book, either directly or indirectly.

Legal Notice:

This book is copyright-protected. It is only for personal use. You cannot amend, distribute, sell, use, quote, or paraphrase any part of the content within this book without the consent of the author or publisher.

Disclaimer Notice:

Please note the information contained within this document is for educational and entertainment purposes only. All efforts have been executed to present accurate, up-to-date, reliable, and complete information. No warranties of any kind are declared or implied. Readers acknowledge that the author is not engaged in the rendering of legal, financial, medical, or professional advice. The content within this book has been derived from various sources. Please consult a licensed professional before attempting any techniques outlined in this book.

By reading this document, the reader agrees that under no circumstances is the author responsible for any losses, direct or indirect, that are incurred as a result of the use of the information contained within this document, including, but not limited to, errors, omissions, or inaccuracies.

WELCOME TO THE WORLD OF THE CARNIVORE INSTINCT! IN A LANDSCAPE OF COUNTLESS DIETARY TRENDS AND FADS, THE CARNIVORE INSTINCT STANDS OUT AS A SIMPLE YET POWERFUL APPROACH TO EATING. BUT WHAT EXACTLY IS THE CARNIVORE INSTINCT, AND WHY HAS IT CAPTURED THE ATTENTION OF SO MANY?

CONTENTS

- 5   INTRODUCTION

PART 1: AWAKENING THE CARNIVORE INSTINCT

- 6   MEAT MADE ME: MY PERSONAL EXPERIENCE
- 7   CHAPTER 1. THE BIRTH OF CARNIVORY: THE EVOLUTION AND PRINCIPLES
- 11   CHAPTER 2. THE POWER OF MEAT: HEALTH BENEFITS AND RISKS
- 15   CHAPTER 3. METABOLIC MAGIC: UNDERSTANDING BODY TRANSFORMATIONS
- 19   CHAPTER 4. CHOOSING THE BEST: QUALITY MEAT AND ETHICAL SOURCING
- 23   CHAPTER 5. EASING INTO CARNIVORY: PRACTICAL TIPS FOR STARTING
- 28   CHAPTER 6. CARNIVORE CLARITY: ANSWERING COMMON QUESTIONS
- 31   CHAPTER 7. REAL-LIFE TRANSFORMATIONS: SUCCESS STORIES

PART 2: CARNIVORE DIET RECIPES

- 34   BREAKFAST
- 47   SNACKS, SIDES, AND SALADS
- 60   BEEF
- 73   PORK
- 86   POULTRY
- 99   SEAFOOD
- 110   OFFAL
- 121   CONCLUSION
- 122   NUTRIENT PROFILES OF ANIMAL-BASED FOODS PER 100 GRAMS
- 128   MEASUREMENT CONVERSIONS
- 130   RECIPE INDEX

INTRODUCTION

WHAT IS THE CARNIVORE INSTINCT?

At its core, the Carnivore Instinct is a way of eating that emphasizes consuming animal foods while excluding plant-based foods. That means no fruits, vegetables, grains, legumes, or other plant-derived products. Instead, the focus is solely on meat, fish, eggs, and other animal products.

BRIEF HISTORY AND ORIGINS OF THE CARNIVORE INSTINCT

While the Carnivore Instinct may seem modern, its roots trace back to our earliest ancestors. For much of human history, our ancestors survived and thrived on diets almost entirely animal foods. It was with the advent of agriculture that humans began incorporating large amounts of plant foods into their diets. In recent years, the Carnivore Diet has experienced a resurgence in popularity thanks to advocates who believe that returning to our ancestral way of eating can lead to numerous health benefits.

WHY THE CARNIVORE INSTINCT?

So why would someone follow the Carnivore Instinct in a world where plant-based diets often take center stage? The reasons are as varied as the individuals who adopt this way of eating. For some, the Carnivore Instinct relieves chronic health conditions like obesity, digestive disorders, and autoimmune diseases. Others are drawn to the simplicity and satiety of a diet based solely on animal foods. And for many, the Carnivore Diet represents a return to a more natural way of eating that feels intuitively right.

OVERVIEW OF WHAT THE BOOK WILL COVER

This book will explore everything you need to know to thrive on the Carnivore Instinct. From understanding the science behind the diet to practical tips for getting started, we'll cover it all. You'll learn how to stock your kitchen with Carnivore-friendly foods, plan satisfying meals, and navigate social situations while staying true to your dietary principles.

Whether you're curious about the Carnivore Diet or ready to dive in headfirst, this book is designed to be your go-to resource for adopting this distinctive approach to eating.

So, grab a steak, sharpen your knives, and embark on this Carnivore journey together!

PART 1: AWAKENING THE CARNIVORE INSTINCT

Dive into the fascinating history and evolution of the carnivore diet and explore the transformation from a plant-heavy lifestyle to embracing our natural meat-eating instincts. This part is your gateway to understanding the core principles of the carnivore diet, enriched with engaging anecdotes and practical tips to kickstart your journey. Let's unravel the secrets of eating like our ancestors and reclaiming your health one juicy steak at a time.

MEAT MADE ME: MY PERSONAL EXPERIENCE

As a kid, I was the picky eater every parent dreads. My diet consisted mostly of PB&Js and the occasional chicken nugget. Vegetables? Only if you counted ketchup. Fast forward a couple of decades, and I found myself donning a chef's hat at the Culinary Institute of America. It was there, amidst the chopping and sizzling, that I began to appreciate the true art of cooking. But little did I know, my culinary journey was about to take a radical turn.

After years of crafting gourmet dishes in some of the finest kitchens across the country, I hit a wall. My health was suffering despite my culinary prowess. I was constantly tired, battling digestive issues, and my weight was creeping up. The irony? I was surrounded by food but felt nutritionally starved.

Enter the carnivore diet. It was a revelation suggested by a fellow chef who had swapped soufflés for steaks and never looked back. At first, the idea of a meat-only diet seemed as alien as a tofu steak. But desperation breeds curiosity, and I decided to give it a go.

My first week was a rollercoaster. I missed my morning croissant, and the thought of another steak made me queasy. But then something incredible happened. I started feeling better. My energy levels soared, my digestion improved, and the weight? It melted away faster than butter in a hot pan.

This newfound vitality ignited a passion in me to delve deeper. I devoured (pun intended) every piece of literature on the carnivore diet, from ancient dietary habits to modern-day success stories. The more I learned, the more I was convinced: this was not just a diet; it was a return to our roots.

Now, I'm here to share my journey and my recipes, crafted with love and a dash of humor. Whether you're a seasoned carnivore or just curious, I hope my story and this cookbook inspire you to explore the carnivore lifestyle. Because if a former veggie-avoider like me can transform his health with a meat-based diet, anyone can. Let's get cooking!

CHAPTER 1.
THE BIRTH OF CARNIVORY: THE EVOLUTION AND PRINCIPLES

Welcome to the first chapter of your carnivore journey! We'll dive into the fascinating history and evolution of the carnivore diet, explore its core principles, and get an up-close look at what it really means to eat like our meat-loving ancestors. Whether you're intrigued by the idea of simplifying your diet or curious about the different ways to embrace this lifestyle, this chapter is your gateway to understanding the delicious, nutritious world of carnivory.

THE HISTORY, EVOLUTION, AND POPULARIZATION

Long before the days of Instagrammable avocado toast and kale smoothies, our ancestors thrived on a simple principle: eat what you can hunt. The life of an ancient hunter-gatherer was anything but easy, yet their diet was as straightforward as it gets—meat, and lots of it. These early humans didn't have food pyramids, but their strength and endurance were proof that they were doing something right.

Fast forward a few millennia, and agriculture changed the game. Suddenly, our plates were overflowing with grains, legumes, and a variety of plants. Diversity in diet seemed like a great idea—until it wasn't. As our diets became more carb-heavy and plant-based, so did our waistlines and our list of chronic illnesses. Who would have thought that the humble potato could be such a troublemaker?

The 20th century brought even more dietary confusion. Fat became the villain, and sugar—well, sugar snuck into everything. Processed foods dominated the market, promising convenience but delivering health issues. Amidst this nutritional chaos, a small group of renegades began to question the status quo. Enter the modern carnivore diet, a radical return to our meat-eating roots.

Dr. Shawn Baker, a prominent figure in the carnivore movement, didn't just talk the talk; he walked the walk—straight to the butcher's counter. His personal transformation and the health benefits he experienced sparked a wave of interest. Suddenly, people everywhere were swapping their salads for steaks, and the results were nothing short of miraculous. Weight loss, increased energy, and mental clarity were just a few of the perks reported by new carnivores.

Of course, no revolutionary idea escapes skepticism. Critics raised concerns about cholesterol and heart disease, but emerging research began to tell a different story. The science supported what our ancestors knew instinctively: meat is not just food; it's fuel.

Today, the carnivore diet is more than a fad; it's a growing movement. People from all walks of life are rediscovering the power of meat-based nutrition. Whether you're here to shed a few pounds, heal chronic conditions, or simply feel better, welcome to the tribe. The carnivore diet isn't just about eating meat; it's about reclaiming your health and reconnecting with a simpler, more natural way of living. So grab a steak, and let's get started!

BASIC PRINCIPLES AND DEFINITION OF THE CARNIVORE DIET

Imagine walking into a restaurant and the menu only has one word: meat. No more debating between the quinoa salad and the gluten-free pasta—just pure, unadulterated, juicy meat. Welcome to the carnivore diet, where simplicity reigns supreme and your only worry is how you want your steak cooked.

The carnivore diet, in its purest form, means eating animal products exclusively. This includes beef, pork, poultry, fish, and organ meats like liver and heart. Eggs and some dairy products can also make the cut, depending on your tolerance. Vegetables, fruits, grains, and all things plant-based are off the table—literally.

But why go to such extremes? The principle behind the carnivore diet is both radical and refreshingly simple: return to our roots. The idea is that our bodies are optimally designed to thrive on animal-based nutrition. This diet eliminates the potential pitfalls of plant-based foods like antinutrients, lectins, and excessive carbohydrates, which can cause inflammation and other health issues.

Think of it as a nutritional cleanse, stripping away all the modern dietary noise and focusing on what our ancestors likely ate. By removing carbs and fiber, the carnivore diet shifts your body into a fat-burning machine, tapping into the clean energy source of ketones. It's like upgrading from regular gasoline to premium—suddenly, you're running smoother and more efficiently.

Critics often gasp at the thought of no veggies, but carnivores are too busy feeling great to care. The benefits reported by those on the diet are impressive: weight loss, improved mental clarity, better digestion, and relief from chronic pain and inflammation. Plus, you get to eat bacon without guilt—how's that for a selling point?

Transitioning to this diet might sound daunting, but it's more intuitive than you'd think. There's no need to count calories or macronutrients. Just eat until you're satisfied, focusing on nutrient-dense, fatty cuts of meat. And if anyone asks why you're skipping the salad, just smile and say, "I'm on a seafood diet—I see food, and I eat it."

In essence, the carnivore diet is about reclaiming a primal way of eating, one that prioritizes simplicity, satiety, and supreme health. It's not just a diet; it's a return to the instincts that once made us strong, resilient, and perfectly adapted to our environment.

LOOK AT THE COMPOSITION OF THE DIET: WHAT FOODS ARE INCLUDED AND WHAT FOODS ARE EXCLUDED

Picture yourself in a grocery store with a mission so simple it's almost laughable: buy meat. Forget the aisles filled with colorful produce, grains, and mysterious health foods with names you can't pronounce. Your shopping list is a carnivore's dream: steak, bacon, chicken, fish, and eggs. It's like a backstage pass to a barbecue festival.

The carnivore diet is built on the foundation of animal-based foods. The stars of this meaty show are beef, pork, lamb, poultry, and fish. Each brings its own set of flavors and nutrients, keeping your palate entertained and your body nourished. Imagine waking up to sizzling bacon and eggs, enjoying a hearty steak for lunch, and finishing your day with a perfectly roasted chicken thigh. It's as if every meal is a celebration of simplicity and flavor.

But the diet isn't just about the main attractions. Organ meats, often called nature's multivitamins, play a crucial role. Liver, kidneys, and heart are nutrient powerhouses packed with vitamins and minerals you won't find in muscle meat. Sure, the idea of eating liver might make you squirm, but sauté it with some butter and spices, and you might just become a believer.

Dairy is another category that can fit into the carnivore lifestyle, depending on individual tolerance. Cheese, butter, and heavy cream can add richness and variety to your meals. Picture a juicy ribeye topped with a pat of melting butter—it's indulgence at its finest.

Now, let's talk about what's left out. This is where the carnivore diet flexes its minimalist muscles. All plant-based foods are excluded. Say goodbye to fruits, vegetables, grains, legumes, nuts, and seeds. No more debating whether kale or spinach is healthier. In the carnivore world, if it didn't have a face or a mother, it's off the menu.

Eliminating these foods might seem restrictive, but it simplifies your diet in a liberating way. You're cutting out potential sources of inflammation and gut irritants found in many plant foods. No more dealing with the hidden sugars in sauces or the sneaky carbs in your "health" snack bars.

By focusing solely on animal products, the carnivore diet streamlines nutrition and maximizes health benefits. It's about returning to the basics, fueling your body with what it's truly designed to process. So, fill your plate with meat, savor every bite, and relish the uncomplicated joy of a carnivore feast. It's not just a diet; it's a deliciously primal way of life.

VARIETIES OF THE CARNIVORE DIET

In the fascinating world of the carnivore diet, there's more than one way to slice a steak. Each variation caters to different health goals, preferences, and lifestyles. Let's explore these diverse paths and find which one might be your perfect match.

The Standard Carnivore Diet

Think of this as the classic approach. The Standard Carnivore Diet focuses predominantly on meat, especially red meats like beef, lamb, and pork. Poultry, fish, and seafood are also welcome, but the emphasis is on consuming fatty cuts to ensure a high intake of natural animal fats. This variant is simple, straightforward, and rich in flavor—perfect for those who love to keep things traditional.

Dairy-Inclusive Carnivore

For the cheese lovers out there, the Dairy-Inclusive Carnivore Diet allows for animal products like cheese, butter, and heavy cream. Incorporating dairy can add a delightful richness to your meals, providing extra fat and nutrients like calcium. However, it's essential to monitor your body's response, as dairy can be a digestive trigger for some.

Whole Animal Carnivore

Going nose-to-tail, this approach encourages eating organ meats and bone broths alongside muscle meats. Liver, heart, and kidneys are rich in nutrients, loaded with essential vitamins and minerals crucial for optimal health. This method not only maximizes nutritional intake but also honors the whole animal, minimizing waste.

High-Fat Carnivore

Designed to mimic ketogenic principles, the High-Fat Carnivore Diet focuses on consuming large amounts of animal fats with moderate protein intake. This variant is particularly popular for weight loss and metabolic health improvements. It emphasizes fatty cuts of meat, lard, and tallow to maintain ketosis and fuel the body efficiently.

Intermittent Fasting with Carnivore

Combining the carnivore diet with intermittent fasting can amplify benefits such as improved insulin sensitivity, weight loss, and mental clarity. This variation involves eating within a restricted time frame—typically an 8-hour window—followed by a 16-hour fast. It's a powerful strategy for those looking to enhance metabolic flexibility and overall health.

Autoimmune Protocol Carnivore

For individuals with autoimmune conditions, this strict form of the carnivore diet eliminates all potential allergens and inflammatory foods, including dairy and eggs. By reducing dietary triggers, this approach aims to manage symptoms and promote gut healing. It's a therapeutic option for those seeking relief from chronic health issues.

Understanding these variations allows you to tailor the carnivore diet to your specific needs, whether you're pursuing weight management, autoimmune support, or simply a sustainable, health-focused lifestyle. Each variant offers unique benefits, and choosing the right one can lead to significant health improvements and culinary satisfaction. So, explore these paths, find your flavor, and embrace the carnivore way!

CHAPTER 2.
THE POWER OF MEAT: HEALTH BENEFITS AND RISKS

In this chapter, we delve into the impressive benefits supported by science. Discover how embracing a meat-based diet can lead to remarkable health improvements while also understanding the potential risks and how to navigate them effectively.

HEALTH BENEFITS, SCIENTIFIC STUDIES AND THERAPEUTIC PROPERTIES OF THE CARNIVORE DIET

The carnivore diet is more than just a culinary choice; it's a powerful tool for transforming your health. This section explores the remarkable benefits supported by scientific studies, from boosting energy and mental clarity to alleviating chronic pain and managing autoimmune diseases. Discover how this meat-centric lifestyle can provide therapeutic benefits, enhancing your overall well-being and vitality.

Boosting Energy Levels and Reducing Fatigue

Starting the day with a hearty steak isn't just a delicious treat; it's a powerful way to fuel your body with sustained energy. One of the most common reports from carnivore dieters is a significant boost in energy levels. Without the blood sugar spikes and crashes caused by carbohydrates, energy remains steady throughout the day. Imagine powering through your tasks with the vigor of a lion on the hunt—sharp, focused, and ready for anything. This consistent energy is thanks to the high protein and fat content of the diet, which provides a slow-burning, efficient fuel source.

Enhancing Mental Clarity and Cognitive Function

Forget the mid-afternoon brain fog. A study published in *Frontiers in Psychology* found that ketogenic diets, which share similarities with the carnivore diet, can enhance cognitive function and reduce brain fog by providing a consistent energy source from ketones. This mental sharpness is attributed to the stable blood sugar levels and the absence of inflammatory compounds found in many plant foods. Think of your brain running on premium fuel, thanks to the high-quality fats and proteins from animal products. No more struggling to remember where you left your keys or what you walked into a room for; instead, you'll be a beacon of clarity and productivity.

Supporting Weight Loss and Metabolic Health

Shedding those extra pounds can feel like an endless battle, but the carnivore diet offers a promising solution. By cutting out carbs and focusing solely on protein and fats, your body enters a state of ketosis, where it burns fat for fuel. This metabolic shift not only aids in weight loss but also helps maintain lean muscle mass. A significant study by Dr. David Ludwig from Harvard Medical School found that low-carb diets like the carnivore diet could boost energy expenditure during weight loss maintenance, making it easier to keep the pounds off. Participants on low-carb diets burned about 200 to 300 more calories per day than those on high-carb diets. Plus, with the high satiety of meat, you'll feel fuller for longer, reducing the temptation to snack on unhealthy foods. It's like having a personal trainer and nutritionist rolled into one, guiding you towards your weight loss goals.

Alleviating Chronic Pain and Inflammation

For those battling chronic pain and inflammation, the carnivore diet can be a game-changer. A study published in the journal *Nutrients* highlighted that low-carb, high-protein diets could reduce markers of inflammation in the body. Many plant foods contain compounds like lectins, phytates and oxalates that can exacerbate inflammation. By eliminating these and focusing on nutrient-dense animal products, inflammation levels can drop significantly. This reduction in inflammation can alleviate symptoms of conditions like arthritis and fibromyalgia. Imagine waking up without the usual aches and pains, ready to tackle the day with newfound ease.

Autoimmune Disease Management

For those battling autoimmune diseases, the carnivore diet can be a beacon of hope. By eliminating most food antigens, which are substances that can trigger immune responses, the diet may help manage and reduce autoimmune symptoms. A study in the *Journal of Clinical Investigation* highlighted that a diet low in potential antigens could reduce the severity of autoimmune conditions like lupus and rheumatoid arthritis. Although more clinical research is needed, many individuals report significant improvements in their symptoms after switching to an all-meat diet.

Improving Digestive Health

While it might seem counterintuitive, removing fiber from the diet can actually improve digestive health for many people. Research indicates that removing fibrous plant materials and other potential irritants allows the digestive system to heal, promoting a more harmonious gut environment. A study in the *World Journal of Gastroenterology* showed that low-fiber diets could improve symptoms in patients with IBS, supporting the benefits observed by carnivore dieters. Your gut becomes a well-oiled machine, processing high-quality proteins and fats efficiently, leading to better digestion and less discomfort.

Stabilizing Mood and Mental Health

Mental health is just as important as physical health, and the carnivore diet can play a crucial role in stabilizing mood and reducing anxiety and depression. The steady energy from fats and proteins supports a balanced release of neurotransmitters, crucial for mood regulation. Additionally, the elimination of sugar and processed foods helps reduce mood swings and irritability. It's like turning your emotional rollercoaster into a calm, steady ride through a serene countryside.

Enhancing Skin Health and Appearance

Your skin is often a reflection of your overall health, and many carnivore dieters notice significant improvements in their skin. Conditions like acne, eczema, and psoriasis can improve or even resolve completely. The high levels of collagen and essential fatty acids in meat contribute to skin elasticity and hydration. Picture yourself with a glowing, clear complexion that radiates health from the inside out.

Supporting Hormonal Balance

Hormones are the body's chemical messengers, and the carnivore diet provides the building blocks needed for their production. A study published in the *Journal of Clinical Endocrinology & Metabolism* found that diets high in saturated fats and low in carbohydrates could boost testosterone levels, which is crucial for both men and women. High-quality animal fats are essential for synthesizing hormones like testosterone and estrogen. This balance is crucial for everything from reproductive health to muscle growth and energy levels. Imagine having the hormonal harmony of a finely-tuned orchestra, each section playing perfectly in sync.

The therapeutic benefits of the carnivore diet extend far beyond weight loss and muscle gain. From enhanced energy and mental clarity to improved digestive health and hormonal balance, this way of eating offers a holistic approach to wellness. By fueling your body with nutrient-dense animal products, you're not just surviving; you're thriving. So next time you dig into a delicious steak, know that you're nourishing your body with everything it needs to perform at its best. Welcome to the carnivore lifestyle, where meat isn't just a meal—it's a pathway to optimal health.

POSSIBLE RISKS AND HOW TO MINIMIZE THEM

Venturing into the carnivore diet can feel like embarking on an exhilarating culinary adventure, but it's crucial to navigate the terrain with your eyes wide open. Just like any diet, the carnivore way comes with its own set of potential pitfalls. Fear not, though—we're here to tackle these risks head-on and arm you with strategies to keep your journey smooth and enjoyable.

Risk: Nutritional Deficiencies

One of the top concerns with a meat-only diet is the potential for missing out on vital nutrients typically found in plant-based foods, such as Vitamin C, fiber, and certain antioxidants.

Solution: Embrace the full spectrum of animal products, especially organ meats like liver and kidney. These are nutritional powerhouses packed with vitamins and minerals. Regularly including a variety of meats and fish can also help cover your nutrient bases. Consider supplements as a safety net—think Vitamin D and omega-3 fatty acids if you're not a fan of fish.

Risk: Heart Disease

Skeptics often raise eyebrows at the idea of consuming large amounts of red meat and saturated fats, worrying about the impact on heart health.

Solution: Focus on quality over quantity. Opt for grass-fed and pasture-raised meats, which have a healthier fat profile. Incorporate fatty fish like salmon, rich in heart-friendly omega-3s. Also, monitor your lipid levels regularly and consult with a healthcare professional to keep your heart health in check.

Risk: Kidney Strain

A high-protein diet can be demanding on the kidneys, especially if pre-existing conditions are a concern.

Solution: Stay hydrated—adequate water intake is crucial to support kidney function. If you have existing kidney issues, it's wise to discuss dietary changes with your doctor. Balance your meat intake with hydration and possibly incorporate more moderate portions of protein-rich foods.

Risk: Digestive Issues

Switching to a carnivore diet can lead to digestive changes, sometimes resulting in constipation due to the lack of dietary fiber.

Solution: Drink plenty of water and include bone broth in your diet, which can help maintain gut health. Adding small amounts of dairy like cheese and yogurt, if tolerated, can also aid digestion. Your body may take time to adjust, so increase your fat intake gradually to help ease the transition.

Risk: Social and Psychological Challenges

Let's face it: eating out and social gatherings can become tricky when you're the only one asking for a steak without the sides.

Solution: Plan ahead. If dining out, check menus in advance or call the restaurant to ensure they can accommodate your preferences. Bring your own meat-based dishes to social events or host gatherings where you can control the menu. Finding online communities or local support groups can also provide motivation and tips for navigating social situations.

Risk: Long-Term Sustainability

The restrictive nature of the carnivore diet raises questions about its long-term sustainability and potential unknown risks over time.

Solution: Approach the diet with flexibility. Periodic medical check-ups are essential to monitor your health. Consider incorporating intermittent fasting or cycling in and out of the strict carnivore diet with phases that include low-carb vegetables. This can help maintain variety and balance while reaping the benefits of a meat-centric diet.

Embarking on the carnivore diet is a bold step towards potentially transformative health benefits, but it's important to proceed with caution and mindfulness. By recognizing these risks and employing thoughtful strategies to mitigate them, you can enjoy the robust advantages of a meat-based diet while maintaining overall well-being. So, gear up with knowledge, listen to your body, and enjoy your carnivore adventure responsibly!

CHAPTER 3.
METABOLIC MAGIC: UNDERSTANDING BODY TRANSFORMATIONS

In this chapter, we'll uncover how the carnivore diet can transform your body from the inside out. Discover how this diet revs up your metabolism, balances your hormones, and optimizes your digestive system. Get ready to understand the physiological magic that happens when you fuel your body with pure, nutrient-dense animal products.

EFFECTS ON METABOLISM AND HORMONAL BALANCE

Imagine your body as a finely-tuned sports car, built for speed and efficiency. Now, what if I told you that by adopting a carnivore diet, you could switch from regular fuel to high-octane performance-enhancing fuel? That's right—let's talk about the turbocharged effects of the carnivore diet on your metabolism and hormonal balance.

When you dive into a meat-only diet, your body undergoes some fascinating transformations. First off, your metabolism gets a serious boost. The carnivore diet is high in protein, and digesting protein requires more energy than fats or carbs—a phenomenon known as the thermic effect of food. This means you're burning more calories just by eating meat. Imagine having a furnace that burns hotter simply because you're fueling it with steak instead of bread.

But it doesn't stop there. By eliminating carbs, your body shifts into ketosis, a metabolic state where fat becomes your primary energy source. It's like flipping a switch from gas to electric—suddenly, you're running on clean, efficient energy. This metabolic shift can lead to significant weight loss and increased energy levels. No more mid-afternoon crashes or cravings for sugary snacks. Instead, you get sustained energy that powers you through the day.

Now, let's talk hormones. The carnivore diet can help balance hormones in remarkable ways. High-quality animal fats and proteins provide the essential building blocks for hormone production. Testosterone, the hormone that fuels muscle growth and vitality, thrives on a diet rich in cholesterol and healthy fats—exactly what you get from meat. Women also benefit as this diet supports balanced estrogen levels, reducing symptoms of hormonal imbalances like PMS and menopause.

The carnivore diet can also positively impact insulin, the hormone that regulates blood sugar levels. Without the constant influx of carbs, your insulin levels stabilize, reducing the risk of insulin resistance and type 2 diabetes. It's like giving your pancreas a well-deserved vacation, allowing it to function more effectively without the constant demand to process sugars.

Ultimately, the carnivore diet transforms your body into a lean, powerful fat-burning machine. It optimizes your metabolism, balances your hormones, and provides a steady source of energy that keeps you at your peak all day long. So, if you're ready to turbocharge your health and feel like a high-performance vehicle, grab that steak and embrace the carnivore lifestyle. It's time to fuel up on the ultimate natural power source.

ADAPTATIONS TO MEAT EATING AND DIGESTIVE HEALTH

Embarking on the carnivore diet is like stepping back into the wild, tapping into ancient instincts that have been dormant for too long. But just as a seasoned hunter knows how to navigate the forest, understanding how our bodies adapt to a meat-based diet can help us thrive in this primal culinary adventure.

When you start eating primarily meat, your digestive system undergoes a fascinating transformation. Initially, you might feel like a novice in the wilderness—unsure, a bit lost, and wondering if you're doing it right. But hang in there; your body is gearing up for a powerful adaptation process.

One of the first things to note is that your stomach becomes a fortress of acidity. The pH level of stomach acid in carnivores is significantly lower, creating an environment that's highly effective at breaking down meat. This heightened acidity not only aids in digestion but also protects against harmful bacteria found in some animal products. It's like your digestive system has upgraded its defenses to match your new diet.

Next, your pancreas steps up its game. Without the need to produce enzymes to break down complex carbohydrates, it focuses on efficiently processing proteins and fats. This shift reduces digestive stress and improves nutrient absorption, making every bite of steak count. Think of it as your pancreas becoming a specialized craftsman, honing its skills to perfection.

Now, let's talk about the gut microbiome. Switching to an all-meat diet significantly alters the microbial landscape of your intestines. While this might sound alarming, it's a natural part of the adaptation. The reduction in fiber means a decrease in certain types of bacteria that thrive on plant matter, but beneficial bacteria that excel at breaking down proteins and fats flourish. This shift can lead to a more stable and less inflammatory gut environment. Imagine your gut flora as a dynamic ecosystem that adjusts to the food you provide—turn it into a well-managed reserve that supports robust health.

In addition to these physical adaptations, your body also becomes more efficient at utilizing fats for energy. This metabolic flexibility means that you can tap into your fat stores more readily, providing a consistent and powerful energy source.

So, as you journey deeper into the carnivore lifestyle, remember that your body is an incredible machine, designed to adapt and thrive. By understanding these adaptations, you can embrace the diet with confidence, knowing that your digestive system is evolving to support your new way of eating. Get ready to unleash your inner carnivore and enjoy the ride—your body's got this!

NUTRITIONAL VALUE OF MEAT AND ANIMAL PRODUCTS

The nutritional value of meat and animal products is a cornerstone of the carnivore diet, providing a powerhouse of essential nutrients that support overall health and well-being. Let's dive into what makes these animal-based foods so remarkable.

Complete Protein Sources

Animal products are considered "complete" proteins because they contain all nine essential amino acids our bodies need. These amino acids are critical for muscle repair, hormone production, and overall cellular function. Unlike plant proteins, which often lack one or more essential amino acids, animal proteins provide a full spectrum, ensuring our bodies can efficiently utilize them for growth and maintenance.

Vitamins

- B Vitamins: Meat, especially red meat and liver, is a rich source of B vitamins, particularly vitamin B12. This vitamin is crucial for nerve function, DNA production, and the formation of red blood cells. Without sufficient B12, you could face serious health issues like anemia and neurological problems.

- Fat-Soluble Vitamins: Vitamins A, D, E, and K are abundant in animal fats. Vitamin A, found in high amounts in liver, supports vision and immune function. Vitamin D, which can be obtained from fatty fish like salmon, is essential for bone health and immune regulation. Vitamin K, present in various animal products, is vital for blood clotting and bone metabolism.

Minerals

Animal products are packed with essential minerals such as iron, zinc, selenium, and magnesium. The iron in meat, known as heme iron, is more easily absorbed by our bodies compared to the non-heme iron found in plant sources. This makes it particularly effective in preventing and treating iron-deficiency anemia. Zinc, abundant in beef and lamb, supports immune function, wound healing, and DNA synthesis.

Fats

- Saturated and Monounsaturated Fats: Animal fats, including those found in beef, pork, and lamb, provide a mix of saturated and monounsaturated fats. These fats are important for maintaining healthy cholesterol levels, supporting brain function, and providing a stable source of energy. Contrary to past misconceptions, moderate consumption of these fats can be part of a healthy diet.

- Omega-3 Fatty Acids: Fatty fish like salmon and mackerel are excellent sources of omega-3 fatty acids, which are crucial for heart health and reducing inflammation. Omega-3s also support brain health, making them a valuable addition to the carnivore diet.

Cholesterol and Other Nutrients

While cholesterol has often been vilified, it plays a crucial role in synthesizing hormones and maintaining cell membranes. The body regulates its own cholesterol production based on dietary intake, meaning that consuming cholesterol-rich foods doesn't necessarily lead to high blood cholesterol levels for most people. Organ meats, such as liver and kidney, also offer a wealth of other nutrients including coenzyme Q10 and alpha-lipoic acid, both of which are important for energy production and antioxidant defense.

Glycine and Collagen

Unique to animal products, glycine and collagen are essential for maintaining healthy skin, joints, and connective tissues. Bone broth, a popular staple in the carnivore diet, is rich in collagen and other joint-supporting compounds like glucosamine and chondroitin. These nutrients help repair tissues and maintain the integrity of our skin and joints.

In conclusion, the nutritional density of meat and animal products makes them an indispensable part of the carnivore diet. They offer a wide array of essential nutrients that support everything from metabolic processes to mental health, highlighting the diet's potential to foster optimal health when high-quality, ethically sourced animal products are chosen.

CHAPTER 4.
CHOOSING THE BEST: QUALITY MEAT AND ETHICAL SOURCING

Choosing the right meat is essential for a successful carnivore journey. This chapter guides you through the landscape of meat selection, from the nutrient-rich benefits of pasture-raised options to the more common grain-fed choices. We'll also explore the importance of organ meats and animal fats, and why sourcing your meat ethically and sustainably matters for both your health and the planet. Dive in to learn how to make the best choices for your carnivore lifestyle, ensuring every bite is as nutritious and ethical as it is delicious.

RECOMMENDATIONS FOR MEAT SELECTION

Selecting the right meat is like choosing a good partner—quality matters, and so does how they've been treated. When embarking on the carnivore diet, your journey begins at the butcher's counter. But don't worry, we're here to guide you through the maze of meat choices.

Pasture-Raised and Grass-Fed

First up, we have the crème de la crème of meats: pasture-raised and grass-fed. Imagine cows grazing freely in lush, green fields under the open sky. This idyllic scene isn't just pleasant; it's the secret to high-quality, nutrient-dense meat. Grass-fed beef boasts higher levels of omega-3 fatty acids, vitamins A and E, and antioxidants like glutathione. Plus, the meat is leaner and the fat it does contain is healthier.

Think of grass-fed beef as the free-range, yoga-practicing, kale-eating supermodel of the meat world. It's pricier, yes, but you're paying for top-notch nutrition and ethical farming practices. When you bite into a grass-fed steak, you're not just tasting the difference—you're savoring a piece of nature's best.

Grain-Fed

Next, we have grain-fed meat. This is the more common and affordable option, where cattle are fed a diet that includes grains like corn and soy. Grain-fed beef tends to be more marbled, with a richer, fattier flavor. It's like the comfort food of the meat world—hearty, satisfying, and readily available.

While grain-fed meat might not have the omega-3 punch of its grass-fed cousin, it still packs a protein punch and can be a staple in your carnivore diet. Just remember, not all grain-fed beef is created equal. Look for labels that ensure the cattle were treated humanely and fed a quality diet without unnecessary antibiotics or hormones.

Organic and Free-Range

Let's not forget about organic and free-range options. Organic meat ensures the animals were raised without synthetic hormones or antibiotics and fed organic feed. Free-range, often associated with poultry, means the animals had some access to the outdoors, which can improve their quality of life and the quality of your meat.

Imagine organic and free-range meat as the eco-friendly, sustainably-sourced option. It's good for you, good for the animal, and good for the planet. If you're conscious about the environmental impact of your diet, this is a great way to align your food choices with your values.

Local and Sustainable

Supporting local farmers who practice sustainable agriculture is another excellent way to ensure you're getting high-quality meat. Visit farmers' markets, join a CSA (Community Supported Agriculture), or even explore local farms. The closer you are to the source, the fresher and more trustworthy your meat will be.

Think of local and sustainable meat as the farm-to-table romance of your carnivore journey. It's fresh, often more flavorful, and helps sustain your local economy. Plus, you get the added bonus of knowing exactly where your food comes from.

Practical Tips for Shopping

When shopping, prioritize cuts that are both nutrient-dense and versatile. Look for fatty cuts like ribeye, brisket, and pork belly, which are rich in flavor and essential nutrients. Don't shy away from offal—liver, kidneys, and heart are nutritional powerhouses.

In summary, choosing the right meat is a blend of quality, ethics, and practicality. Whether you opt for grass-fed luxury or grain-fed comfort, what matters most is how you prepare and enjoy it. So, happy hunting!

THE ROLE OF ORGAN MEATS AND ANIMAL FATS

If you're diving into the carnivore diet, get ready to embrace the unsung heroes of the animal kingdom: organ meats and animal fats. These nutritional powerhouses are not only delicious but also packed with essential vitamins and minerals that your body craves.

Organ Meats: Nature's Multivitamins

Organ meats like liver, kidneys, and heart are often overlooked, but they're incredibly nutrient-dense. Think of them as nature's multivitamins. Liver, for instance, is a superstar, loaded with vitamins A, D, E, K, B12, and folic acid, along with essential minerals like iron and copper. These nutrients play crucial roles in everything from boosting your immune system to enhancing brain health.

But let's be honest, the idea of eating organ meats can be a bit daunting at first. The trick is to ease into it. Start with small quantities, perhaps mixed into ground beef. Over time, you might find yourself actually looking forward to liver night. And if you're still hesitant, try making a delicious liver pâté—smooth, flavorful, and perfect for spreading on your favorite meat.

The Mighty Animal Fats

Now, onto the fats. Animal fats like tallow, lard, and butter are essential on the carnivore diet. They provide a rich source of energy and are crucial for absorbing fat-soluble vitamins like A, D, E, and K. Plus, they add incredible flavor to your dishes.

For years, fats have been unfairly demonized, but we're here to set the record straight. Saturated fats are not the enemy; in fact, they play a vital role in hormone production and maintaining cell integrity. Monounsaturated fats, particularly from sources like lard and tallow, can even improve cardiovascular health when consumed in moderation.

Cooking with Animal Fats

One of the best things about animal fats is their stability at high temperatures. Unlike many vegetable oils, which can oxidize and create harmful compounds when heated, animal fats remain stable. This makes them ideal for frying, and roasting. Plus, they impart a depth of flavor that's hard to beat.

Incorporating these elements into your diet can seem challenging at first, but with a bit of culinary creativity and an open mind, you'll soon discover a world of rich flavors and unparalleled nutrition. So, go ahead and give organ meats and animal fats a try—they might just become your new favorites on this carnivore journey.

ETHICAL AND SUSTAINABLE SOURCES OF MEAT

In the world of carnivore dining, it's not just about the meat on your plate but also about where it comes from. Ethical and sustainable meat sourcing isn't just a trend—it's a crucial component of responsible eating that benefits your health, the environment, and the animals. So, let's discover how to make conscious choices without sacrificing taste.

The Ethics of Eating Meat

Picture this: lush green pastures, cows grazing freely, chickens pecking around happily, and pigs wallowing in mud. Sounds idyllic, right? That's because it is. Ethical meat comes from animals that are treated humanely, allowed to exhibit natural behaviors, and raised without unnecessary antibiotics or hormones. It's about respecting the animals and ensuring they lead good lives before they become part of our diet.

Sustainable Farming Practices

Sustainability in meat production goes hand-in-hand with ethical farming. Sustainable farms focus on regenerative practices that replenish the land, reduce carbon footprints, and promote biodiversity. This includes rotational grazing, where animals are moved between pastures to prevent overgrazing and encourage soil health. It's like giving the land a well-deserved spa day, helping it rejuvenate and support future generations of livestock.

Choosing the Right Sources

When shopping for meat, look for labels like "grass-fed," "pasture-raised," and "organic." Organic meats ensure no synthetic pesticides or genetically modified organisms (GMOs) are used, and antibiotics are only administered when necessary.

Buying directly from local farmers or farmers' markets can also ensure you're getting high-quality meat. It's like having a direct line to the source, where you can ask about their farming practices, see the conditions, and often even meet the animals. Plus, supporting local farms helps boost your local economy and reduce the carbon footprint associated with transporting food over long distances.

The Impact on Your Plate and Beyond

Ethically sourced and sustainably raised meat doesn't just taste better—it's better for you and the planet. Animals that roam freely and eat natural diets are healthier, and their meat reflects that quality. You get fewer harmful residues and more nutrients. Plus, knowing that your food choices are supporting good practices can make every meal feel a bit more fulfilling.

By choosing meat from ethical and sustainable sources, you're also helping combat some of the negative impacts of industrial farming, such as soil degradation, water pollution, and greenhouse gas emissions. It's a small step towards a larger goal of creating a more balanced and respectful relationship with our food and the planet.

Practical Tips for Ethical Eating

Start by researching local farms and butchers committed to ethical practices. Online resources and farm directories can be invaluable. Also, don't be afraid to ask questions—whether you're at a farmers' market or a grocery store. Transparency is key to making informed choices.

In the grand tapestry of the carnivore diet, ethical and sustainable meat sourcing is a vibrant thread that enhances the whole experience. It's about enjoying delicious, nutrient-dense foods while honoring the animals and the earth. So, next time you fire up the grill, take pride in knowing that your meal is as kind to the planet as it is satisfying to your taste buds. Happy ethical eating!

CHAPTER 5.
EASING INTO CARNIVORY: PRACTICAL TIPS FOR STARTING

Starting the carnivore diet can feel like stepping into a new, meat-filled world, but with the right tips and mindset, the transition can be smooth and rewarding. This chapter provides practical advice on easing into the diet, overcoming initial challenges, and handling social situations with confidence and humor. Let's make your journey to carnivory as enjoyable and successful as possible!

PRACTICAL TIPS FOR TRANSITIONING TO THE CARNIVORE DIET

Transitioning to the carnivore diet might seem as intimidating as stepping into a world where vegetables are outlawed and meat reigns supreme. But fear not, dear reader! With the right mindset and a few practical tips, you'll find this journey as satisfying as biting into a perfectly seared steak. Let's get you started on the right hoof!

Start Slowly, But Start Now

Going full carnivore overnight can be a shock to your system, especially if you've been living on salads and smoothies. Begin by gradually reducing your intake of carbs and plant-based foods while increasing your consumption of meat and animal products. Think of it as wading into a pool rather than diving headfirst. Swap your usual breakfast cereal for bacon and eggs, replace your lunchtime sandwich with a hearty steak, and make dinner all about that juicy pork chop.

Stock Up on Essentials

Preparation is key. Stock your kitchen with a variety of meats, including beef, pork, chicken, and fish. Don't forget organ meats like liver and heart—they're nutrient powerhouses. Also, keep a good supply of animal fats like tallow, lard, and butter for cooking. Having a well-stocked fridge and pantry will make it easier to stay on track and resist the temptation to reach for non-carnivore snacks.

Embrace Simplicity

One of the beauties of the carnivore diet is its simplicity. Meals are straightforward and require minimal preparation. Grill, roast, or pan-fry your meat with a sprinkle of salt, and you're good to go. If you're feeling adventurous, experiment with different cuts and cooking methods, but remember, the focus is on enjoying the natural flavors of the meat.

Listen to Your Body

Your body knows best. As you transition, pay attention to how you feel. Some people experience what's known as the "keto flu"—a temporary phase of fatigue and headaches as your body adjusts to burning fat for fuel. Stay hydrated, ensure you're getting enough electrolytes (like sodium, potassium, and magnesium), and give yourself time to adapt. If you feel hungry, eat. If you feel full, stop. The carnivore diet is about listening to your body's signals and responding intuitively.

Social Situations and Dining Out

Social gatherings and dining out can be tricky, but they're manageable with a bit of planning. When eating out, choose restaurants that serve quality meat dishes. Don't hesitate to ask for modifications. At social events, offer to bring a meat-based dish to share, ensuring you have something you can enjoy. Remember, confidence is key. Explain your dietary choices briefly if asked, but don't feel pressured to justify your lifestyle.

Celebrate Small Wins

Transitioning to a new diet is a big deal, and it's important to celebrate your progress. Each successful meal, each day you stick to the plan, is a victory. Keep a journal or share your journey with friends or online communities. Celebrate the milestones—whether it's improved energy, better digestion, or simply feeling great about what you're eating.

By starting slowly, stocking up on essentials, embracing simplicity, listening to your body, navigating social situations with confidence, and celebrating your progress, you'll find that transitioning to the carnivore diet can be a rewarding and enjoyable experience. So, get ready to cook up a storm, enjoy every bite, and embrace the carnivore lifestyle—where eating meat becomes a rewarding and fulfilling habit.

INITIAL DIFFICULTIES AND HOW TO OVERCOME THEM

Switching to the carnivore diet can feel like you've traded your comfy slippers for a pair of hiking boots. The path ahead is exciting, but it might have a few bumps. Don't worry—every challenge has a solution, and soon you'll be navigating this new lifestyle with confidence.

The "Keto Flu"

Many newcomers experience the so-called "keto flu" during the first week. Symptoms like fatigue, headaches, and irritability are common as your body adapts from burning carbs to burning fat for fuel. Think of it as a mini-detox. To ease this transition, stay hydrated, add a pinch of salt to your water, and ensure you're getting enough electrolytes. Bone broth is your best friend here—it's packed with minerals and can help you feel better faster.

Cravings for Carbs and Sugars

Missing your favorite carb-loaded snacks? You're not alone. Cravings can hit hard, especially in the beginning. Combat them by focusing on nutrient-dense, satisfying meats. Keep a stash of quick, protein-rich snacks like beef jerky or hard-boiled eggs. Sometimes, cravings are more about habit than hunger, so keep busy and stay focused on your goals. Over time, your taste buds will adjust, and those cravings will fade.

Digestive Adjustments

Your digestive system might need some time to get used to an all-meat diet. You might experience changes in bowel movements, from constipation to diarrhea. To help your gut adapt, increase your intake of fat gradually and make sure you're drinking plenty of water. Incorporating bone broth can also soothe your digestive tract and promote healthy gut function. If issues persist, try including small amounts of dairy or eggs to see if they help.

Eating Out and On-the-Go

Dining out while sticking to the carnivore diet might seem daunting, but it's entirely doable. Choose restaurants that specialize in grilled meats or seafood. Don't hesitate to ask for modifications—most chefs are happy to accommodate dietary needs. When traveling or on-the-go, pack some portable snacks. Planning ahead ensures you always have carnivore-friendly options at hand.

Dealing with Boredom

Eating meat every day might sound repetitive, but it doesn't have to be boring. Explore different cuts of meat, experiment with various cooking methods, and try new seasonings. From a slow-cooked brisket to a quick seared tuna steak, the possibilities are endless. Keeping your meals varied and flavorful will keep your palate entertained and your diet sustainable.

Energy Slumps

Some people might feel an initial drop in energy levels. This is usually temporary as your body adjusts to its new fuel source. Make sure you're eating enough fat and getting plenty of rest. Gradually, you'll notice a steady increase in energy and endurance. Remember, this is a marathon, not a sprint.

Embracing the carnivore diet is a journey, and like any journey, it has its challenges. By staying informed and prepared, you can overcome these initial difficulties with ease. Stick with it, and you'll find that the benefits far outweigh the bumps along the way. So keep your spirits high, and enjoy every step of your carnivore adventure.

MANAGING SOCIAL SITUATIONS AND DIETARY CHALLENGES

Embarking on the carnivore diet can feel like you've become a culinary maverick in a world full of plant-eaters. Navigating social situations with your new meat-focused lifestyle can be tricky, but it's entirely possible with a bit of planning, a touch of confidence, and a dash of humor. Let's dive into some practical tips to help you manage social situations and dietary challenges without compromising your dietary goals or your social life.

Be Open and Honest

When it comes to social gatherings, transparency is your best ally. Let your friends and family know about your dietary choices upfront. You don't need to deliver a TED Talk on the benefits of the carnivore diet—unless you want to—but a brief, honest explanation can go a long way. You might say something like, "I'm following a meat-based diet for health reasons, so I'll be focusing on the meat dishes tonight." This openness not only sets expectations but can also spark curiosity and support.

Scout the Menu

Dining out doesn't have to be a nightmare. Before heading to a restaurant, check the menu online or give them a call to see if they can accommodate your needs. Steakhouses, barbecue joints, and seafood restaurants are typically safe bets. Don't hesitate to ask for modifications; most places are happy to grill up a plain steak or a piece of fish without the carb-laden sides. Remember, you're the customer, and your dietary needs are important.

Bring Your Own Meat

If you're attending a potluck or a family gathering, offer to bring a meat dish. Not only does this ensure you have something delicious to eat, but it also introduces others to the tasty possibilities of the carnivore diet. Think of it as a delicious way to share your new lifestyle with loved ones. Whether it's a platter of juicy meatballs or a slow-cooked brisket, your contribution will likely be a hit.

Focus on Fun, Not Food

At social events, try shifting the focus from food to fun. Engage in conversations, participate in activities, and enjoy the company. When the emphasis is on the social aspects of the gathering, the food becomes secondary. Plus, your enthusiasm and positive energy can be contagious, making the event enjoyable for everyone, regardless of what's on their plate.

Handle Criticism with Grace

Not everyone will understand or agree with your dietary choices, and that's okay. When faced with criticism or curious questions, respond calmly and confidently. Share the positive changes you've experienced and the reasons behind your choice. Sometimes, your personal story can be more compelling than any scientific argument. And if the discussion gets too intense, it's perfectly fine to change the subject with a light-hearted comment or a joke.

Holidays and Special Occasions

Holidays can be particularly challenging due to their food-centric nature. Plan ahead by preparing carnivore-friendly versions of holiday favorites or focusing on the meat dishes that are already part of the tradition. Offering to host can also give you more control over the menu. Remember, the goal is to enjoy the time with your loved ones, not to stress over every bite.

Stay Connected

Join online forums or local groups of fellow carnivores. Sharing experiences, tips, and encouragement with like-minded individuals can be incredibly supportive. Knowing you're not alone in your journey can boost your confidence and provide you with practical advice for navigating social scenarios.

By being prepared, staying flexible, and maintaining a positive attitude, you can enjoy a vibrant social life while adhering to your carnivore diet. Remember, it's all about balance and making choices that align with your health goals without isolating yourself from the joy of shared meals and experiences. Happy socializing!

CHAPTER 6.
CARNIVORE CLARITY: ANSWERING COMMON QUESTIONS

When adopting the carnivore diet, individuals often face a myriad of questions from themselves and curious friends and family. This chapter addresses the most common questions, providing clear and concise answers to help you navigate your carnivore journey more effectively.

---

1. How Do I Start the Carnivore Diet?

Embarking on the carnivore diet is like jumping into a meaty adventure. Start by gradually reducing plant-based foods and increasing your intake of animal products. Begin with the basics: beef, lamb, pork, and poultry. Over time, introduce organ meats and fish. Plan your meals, keep it simple, and remember: consistency is key. Your body will thank you for the transition with newfound energy and vitality.

2. What Can I Eat on the Carnivore Diet?

The carnivore diet is all about keeping it straightforward: if it's from an animal, it's on the menu. This includes all types of meat, fish, eggs, and animal-derived products like lard and bone broth. Dairy is also acceptable, particularly high-fat options like butter and cream. Imagine a world where bacon is your bread and ribeyes are your vegetables—paradise, right?

3. How Much to Eat and How Often on a Carnivore Diet?

Eat when you're hungry and stop when you're full. It's that simple. Initially, you might find yourself eating more frequently as your body adjusts. Eventually, many people find they need fewer meals per day because the diet is incredibly satiating. Listen to your body's signals, and don't be afraid to indulge in that second steak if you're still hungry.

4. Can I Drink Tea or Coffee on the Carnivore Diet?

Yes, you can! Most carnivore dieters enjoy coffee and tea, but be mindful of additives. Stick to black coffee and plain tea to keep it pure and simple. If you're a fan of frothy lattes, try using heavy cream instead of milk to stay true to the high-fat, low-carb ethos.

5. Can I Eat Dairy on the Carnivore Diet?

Dairy can be a part of your carnivore journey, especially if you tolerate it well. Opt for high-fat options like butter, cream, and cheese. Remember, each body is different, so pay attention to how dairy affects you. If you notice any digestive discomfort, it might be worth experimenting with reducing or eliminating it.

6. Can You Eat Processed Meats Like Sausage and Deli Meat on the Carnivore Diet?

Processed meats can be included but with caution. Look for products with minimal additives, ideally just meat and seasoning. Avoid those with sugars, fillers, and preservatives. Your local butcher can be a great resource for high-quality, minimally processed options.

7. Do I Need Carbohydrates on the Carnivore Diet?

Nope! The carnivore diet is all about ditching carbs. Your body can efficiently run on fats and proteins, entering a state called ketosis where fat becomes your primary fuel source. This not only helps in weight loss but also provides steady energy levels and mental clarity.

8. Can I Exercise on the Carnivore Diet?

Absolutely! Many carnivores report improved performance and recovery times once their bodies adapt. Initially, you might experience some fatigue as your body shifts to burning fat for fuel. Stay hydrated, ensure adequate electrolyte intake, and soon you'll find yourself running circles around your old self at the gym.

9. How Do I Get Vitamins and Minerals Without Fruits and Vegetables?

Imagine getting all your nutrients from a juicy steak. Yes, it's possible! Meat, particularly organ meats like liver, is nutrient-dense and packed with essential vitamins and minerals. You'll get your vitamin C from liver, magnesium from beef, and omega-3s from fatty fish. Think of it as nature's multivitamin, but way tastier. Just ensure you're eating a variety of meats to cover all your nutritional bases.

10. Is the Carnivore Diet Safe During Pregnancy?

Eating for two the carnivore way can be safe and beneficial, but it's crucial to consult with your healthcare provider first. Many women find that a high-protein, nutrient-dense diet supports their energy levels and overall health during pregnancy. Focus on including a variety of meats, especially nutrient-rich organ meats, to provide essential nutrients for both you and your baby.

11. Is It Necessary to Take Supplements on the Carnivore Diet?

While a well-rounded carnivore diet can provide most of the nutrients you need, some people might benefit from supplements. Common ones include electrolytes (sodium, potassium, magnesium) and possibly vitamin D if you're not getting enough sunlight. Listen to your body and consider getting blood work done to check for any deficiencies. Supplements can be a helpful safety net, but they're not a mandatory part of the carnivore life.

12. How Do You Go to the Bathroom Without Fiber on the Carnivore Diet?

Contrary to popular belief, your bathroom routine won't be ruined without fiber. Many carnivores report improved digestion and less frequent bowel movements. Meat is highly digestible, and the absence of fiber can reduce bloating and gas. Stay hydrated, and if you encounter issues, a bit of magnesium or more fat in your diet can help keep things moving smoothly.

13. What Are the Differences Between the Keto and Carnivore Diets?

Both diets are low-carb, but the carnivore diet takes it to the next level by eliminating all plant foods. Keto allows for a variety of low-carb vegetables, nuts, and seeds, whereas carnivore sticks strictly to animal products. Think of keto as the less strict older sibling and carnivore as the hardcore minimalist. Both can help with weight loss and improved health, but carnivore is the ultimate elimination diet.

14. What Are the Benefits of the Carnivore Diet Over Plant-Based Diets?

The carnivore diet focuses on simplicity and nutrient density. By cutting out plant foods, you eliminate potential sources of antinutrients and digestive irritants. Meat is a complete protein source, rich in bioavailable nutrients that are easy for your body to absorb. Additionally, many find they have more stable energy levels, better mental clarity, and fewer cravings on a carnivore diet compared to plant-based diets.

15. What Are the Common Side Effects During the Adaptation Phase?

The transition to carnivore can come with a few bumps, known as the "carnivore flu." You might experience fatigue, headaches, and irritability as your body adapts to burning fat for fuel. Hydration and electrolytes are your best friends during this phase. Most people find these symptoms subside within a few weeks, leaving them feeling better than ever.

16. How Long Does It Take to See Results?

Patience! Some people notice benefits like increased energy and reduced cravings within days. For more significant changes, like weight loss and improved mental clarity, give it a few weeks to a few months. Everyone's body is different, but with consistency, you'll start seeing and feeling the benefits of your carnivore journey.

Embarking on the carnivore diet might seem daunting at first, but with these answers in hand, you're well on your way to mastering this meat-centric lifestyle. Keep your approach simple, listen to your body, and enjoy the journey back to your natural eating instincts.

CHAPTER 7.
REAL-LIFE TRANSFORMATIONS: SUCCESS STORIES

The carnivore diet, while scientifically intriguing, comes to life through the stories of those who have embraced it. This chapter compiles a series of testimonials and success stories from individuals who have experienced profound transformations in their health, well-being, and overall lifestyle by adopting this all-meat regimen.

---

1. Overcoming Chronic Health Issues:

John, a 45-year-old with a history of Type 2 diabetes and obesity, struggled with managing his blood sugar levels despite various diets. After switching to a carnivore diet, John reported a significant decrease in his blood sugar levels, reduced medication dependency, and a weight loss of 50 pounds over six months. His energy levels increased, allowing him to enjoy activities he had avoided for years.

2. Improved Mental Clarity and Mood:

Sarah, a 35-year-old freelance writer, suffered from frequent migraines and brain fog, which impacted her ability to work. Within weeks of starting the carnivore diet, she noticed a clear improvement in her cognitive functions, cessation of migraines, and an uplift in her mood and productivity.

3. Digestive Health Transformation:

Alex, a 30-year-old software developer, had chronic irritable bowel syndrome (IBS) that interfered with his daily life. The switch to a carnivore diet eliminated his bloating and unpredictable bowel habits. Alex shared that this change allowed him to lead a normal life without the constant worry about his digestive issues.

4. Athletic Performance and Recovery:

Emily, a competitive athlete, adopted the carnivore diet to optimize her performance and recovery times. She experienced increased muscle mass, improved stamina, and faster recovery between training sessions. Emily's coaches and teammates noted her enhanced ability to perform at high levels consistently.

5. Autoimmune Relief:

Mark, who dealt with rheumatoid arthritis, embarked on a carnivore diet after other treatments failed to ease his pain significantly. Months into the diet, Mark experienced a dramatic reduction in joint pain and inflammation, attributing this improvement to the elimination of inflammatory plant foods.

6. Longevity and Sustained Health:

Helen, a 67-year-old retiree, turned to the carnivore diet to improve her general health. A year later, she reports better mobility, fewer age-related health issues, and a more active lifestyle, suggesting that the diet may have benefits for aging populations seeking to maintain their health and vitality.

7. Improved Skin Conditions:

Lisa, a 28-year-old graphic designer, struggled with severe acne for years. After multiple unsuccessful treatments, she switched to a carnivore diet. Within a few months, Lisa reported a significant improvement in her skin clarity. She believes the elimination of sugar and processed foods played a critical role in reducing her skin inflammation.

8. Enhanced Mental Well-being:

Tom, a 42-year-old teacher, experienced chronic depression and anxiety. Seeking a change after traditional therapies provided limited relief, he adopted a carnivore diet. Tom noted a marked improvement in his mood and energy levels, attributing this change to the stabilizing effects of the diet on his blood sugar and hormonal balance.

9. Resolution of Digestive Disorders:

Anita, a 34-year-old nurse, suffered from Crohn's disease, which frequently disrupted her ability to work. After transitioning to a carnivore diet, Anita experienced a dramatic decrease in gastrointestinal symptoms, allowing her to manage her condition more effectively without reliance on frequent medication.

10. Sustained Weight Loss:

Derek, a 50-year-old business owner, battled with obesity and high blood pressure. On his doctor's advice, he switched to a carnivore diet, focusing on lean meats and avoiding processed foods. Over a year, Derek lost over 70 pounds and saw a significant improvement in his blood pressure and overall cardiovascular health.

These stories represent a spectrum of personal health journeys and outcomes on the carnivore diet. While not universally applicable, these testimonials highlight potential benefits and encourage a personalized approach to nutrition. For anyone considering the carnivore diet, these success stories offer insight and inspiration, showcasing the transformative power of dietary change in achieving health and wellness goals. Each story underscores the importance of careful consideration, consultation with health professionals, and mindful monitoring when embarking on such a significant dietary shift.

PART 2:
CARNIVORE DIET RECIPES

Step into the kitchen where meat reigns supreme! This part is packed with mouthwatering recipes that cater to every carnivore's palate. From sizzling breakfasts to hearty dinners, discover the joy of crafting delicious, nutrient-dense meals that are both simple and satisfying. Whether you're a seasoned carnivore or new to this lifestyle, these recipes will fuel your body and excite your taste buds, proving that a meat-based diet can be diverse, flavorful, and downright fun.

BREAKFAST

35	BEEF AND EGG SCRAMBLE
36	CREAMY SCRAMBLED EGGS
37	EGG AND SHRIMP BAKE
38	PORK RIND PANCAKES
39	BONE MARROW WITH FRIED EGGS
40	BACON-WRAPPED EGGS WITH SOFT CHEESE
41	EGG MUFFINS
42	BEEF OMELET
43	SAUSAGE SCRAMBLE
44	CARNIVORE BREAKFAST PIZZA
45	CHEESE-CRUSTED HAM AND EGG SANDWICH
46	CARNIVORE DIET BREAKFAST TACOS

BEEF AND EGG SCRAMBLE

SERVING 2
PREP TIME: 5 MIN
COOK TIME: 15 MIN

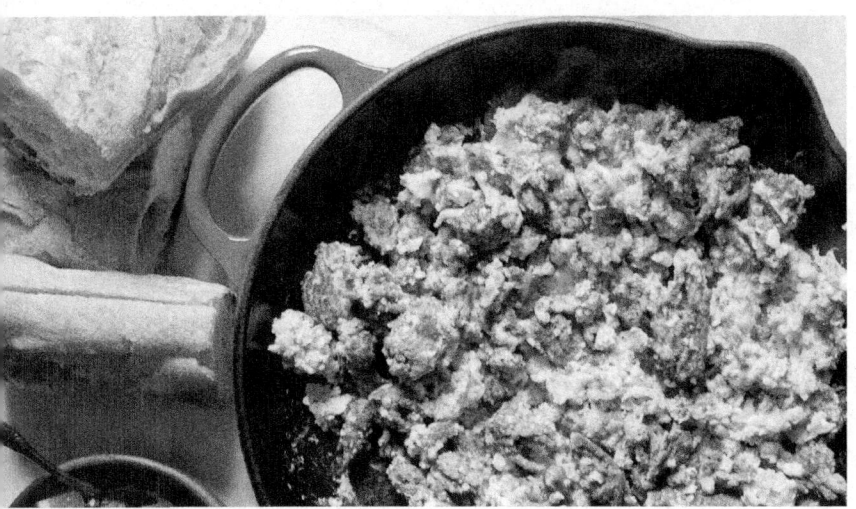

This hearty breakfast dish combines ground beef and eggs, offering a protein-packed start to your day. Quick to prepare, it delivers savory flavors with minimal effort.

INGREDIENTS

- Drizzle beef tallow
- 1/2 lb ground beef
- 4 large eggs
- Salt, to taste
- Freshly ground black pepper (as much as preferred)

INSTRUCTIONS

1. Heat a drizzle of avocado oil or beef tallow in a skillet over medium heat.
2. Cook the ground beef in a skillet until it's fully browned and cooked through, which should take approximately 7 to 10 minutes.
3. In a small bowl, whisk the eggs together with a pinch of salt and black pepper.
4. Transfer the beaten eggs to the skillet containing the cooked ground beef.
5. Feel free to keep stirring until the eggs are entirely cooked and scrambled, typically around 3 to 5 minutes.

NUTRITIONAL INFO

Cal 300 • Fat 20 g • Carb 0 g • Protein 30 g

ALLERGEN INFO

CREAMY SCRAMBLED EGGS

SERVING 2
PREP TIME: 5 MIN
COOK TIME: 5 MIN

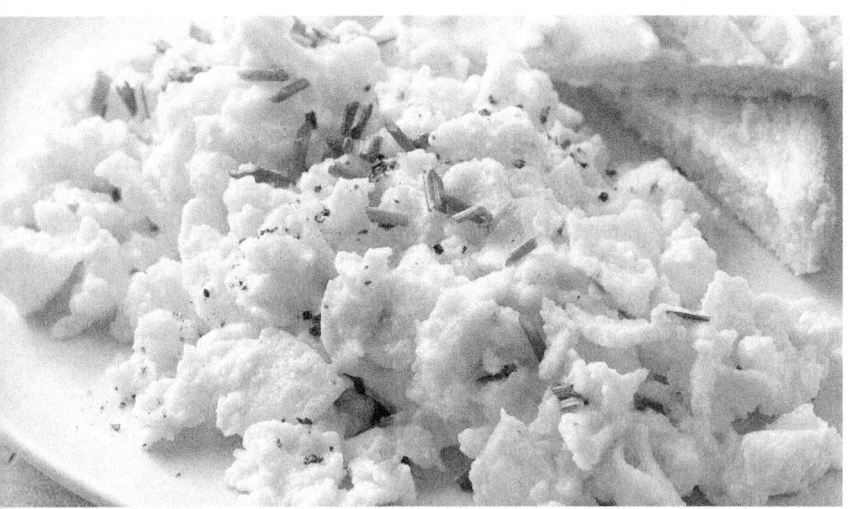

Indulge in these rich and creamy scrambled eggs, enhanced with heavy cream, for a velvety texture. They're perfect for a quick and enjoyable breakfast.

INGREDIENTS

- 6 large eggs
- 2 tablespoons heavy cream
- Salt, to taste
- Freshly ground black pepper (as much as preferred)
- 1 tablespoon butter

NUTRITIONAL INFO

Cal 280 • Fat 22 g • Carb 1 g • Protein 18 g

ALLERGEN INFO

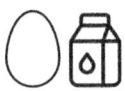

INSTRUCTIONS

1. Crack the eggs into a mixing bowl. Add heavy cream, salt, and pepper. Whisk until well combined.
2. Melt the butter in a skillet.
3. Pour the egg mixture into the skillet.
4. Using a spatula, gently stir the eggs as they cook.
5. Cook until the eggs are creamy and slightly runny, about 3–5 minutes.
6. Remove from heat and serve immediately.

EGG AND SHRIMP BAKE

SERVING 2
PREP TIME: 5 MIN
COOK TIME: 20 MIN

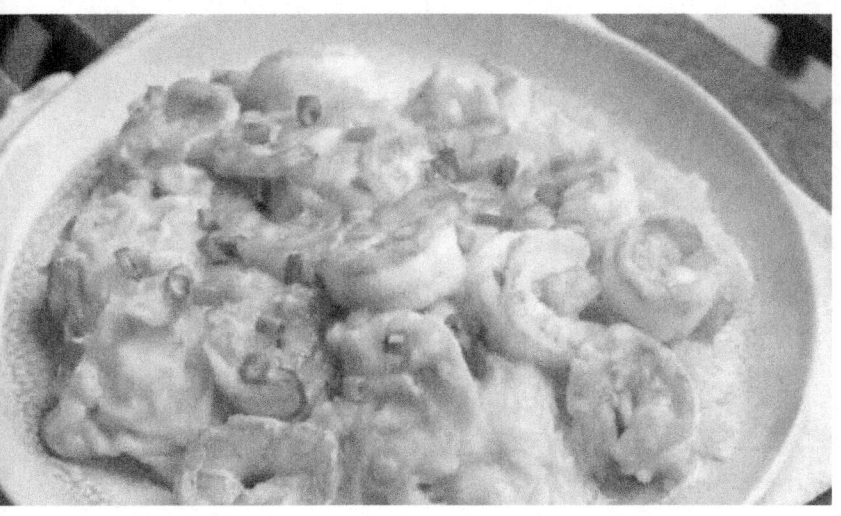

This oven-baked dish features a delightful combination of shrimp and eggs, creating a luxurious yet simple breakfast option. It's an excellent way to enjoy seafood first thing in the morning.

INGREDIENTS

- 4 large eggs
- 1/2 lb shrimp, peeled and deveined
- Salt, to taste
- Freshly ground black pepper (as much as preferred)
- 1 tablespoon of butter

NUTRITIONAL INFO

Cal 320 • Fat 20 g • Carb 2 g • Protein 30 g

ALLERGEN INFO

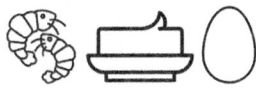

INSTRUCTIONS

1. Commence by raising the oven's temperature to 375°F (190°C).
2. Grease a small baking dish with butter.
3. Arrange the shrimp evenly in the baking dish.
4. Crack the eggs over the shrimp.
5. Season with salt and pepper.
6. Bake in the oven until the eggs are set, and the shrimp are cooked for 15-20 minutes.
7. After removing it from the oven, let the dish cool for a while before serving.

BREAKFAST

PORK RIND PANCAKES

SERVING 2
PREP TIME: 5 MIN
COOK TIME: 20 MIN

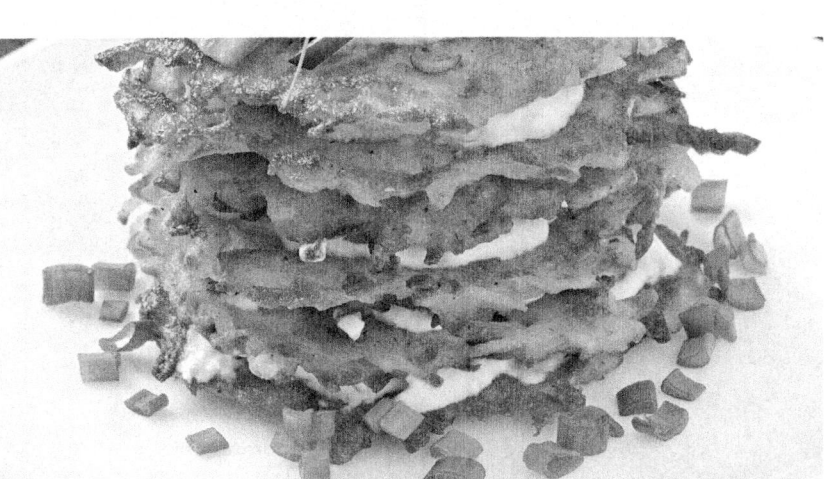

These crispy pancakes from crushed pork rinds are a unique carnivore twist on a breakfast classic. Enjoy them plain or with your favorite carnivore-friendly toppings.

INGREDIENTS

- 1 cup pork rinds, crushed
- 2 large eggs
- 2 tablespoons heavy cream
- Salt, to taste
- 2 tablespoons butter or bacon grease

NUTRITIONAL INFO

Cal 240 • Fat 18 g • Carb 0 g • Protein 20 g

ALLERGEN INFO

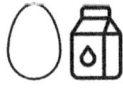

INSTRUCTIONS

1. Combine crushed pork rinds, eggs, heavy cream, and salt in a mixing bowl. Mix until well combined.
2. Before you start, heat a skillet over medium heat and then melt the butter or bacon grease in it.
3. Scoop the pancake batter onto the skillet, shaping small pancakes.
4. Cook until golden brown on both sides, about 2-3 minutes per side.
5. Serve hot with your favorite carnivore-friendly toppings, or enjoy them as they are.

BONE MARROW
WITH FRIED EGGS

SERVING 2
PREP TIME: 5 MIN
COOK TIME: 20 MIN

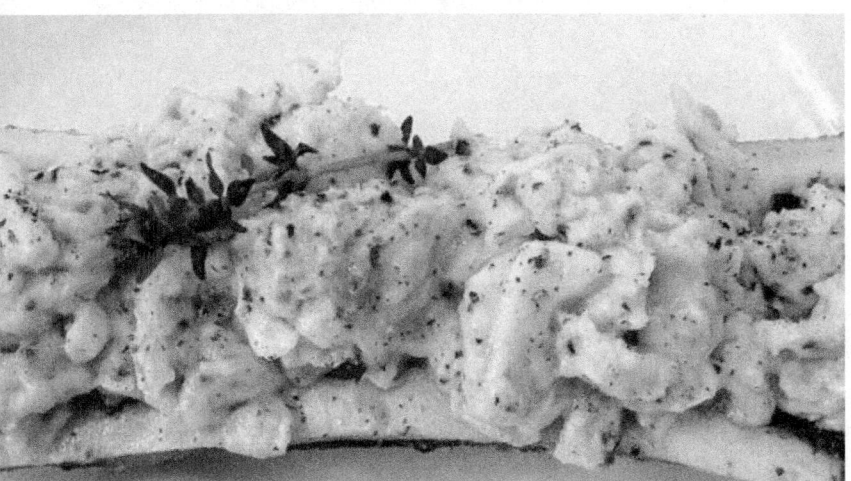

A decadent breakfast featuring roasted bone marrow served with perfectly fried eggs. This dish is rich in nutrients and offers an indulgent start to your day.

INGREDIENTS

- 2 beef marrow bones, cut lengthwise
- 4 large eggs
- Salt, to taste
- Freshly ground black pepper (as much as preferred)
- Drizzle beef tallow

NUTRITIONAL INFO

Cal 450 • Fat 40 g • Carb 0 g • Protein 20 g

ALLERGEN INFO

INSTRUCTIONS

1. Commence by preheating the oven to 400°F (200°C).
2. To prepare, put the marrow bones on a baking sheet (the cut side upwards). Drizzle with beef tallow.
3. Roast in the oven until the marrow is soft and bubbly, about 15-20 minutes.
4. While the bones are roasting, warm a skillet over medium heat.
5. Crack the eggs in a skillet and fry until the whites are cooked through, but the yolks remain runny, typically for about 3-4 minutes.
6. Season the eggs with salt and pepper.
7. After the marrow bones have finished cooking, take them out of the oven and let them cool down for a bit.
8. Serve the roasted marrow bones with the fried eggs on top.
9. Optionally, sprinkle with additional salt and pepper to taste.

BACON-WRAPPED EGGS
WITH SOFT CHEESE

SERVING 2
PREP TIME: 5 MIN
COOK TIME: 20 MIN

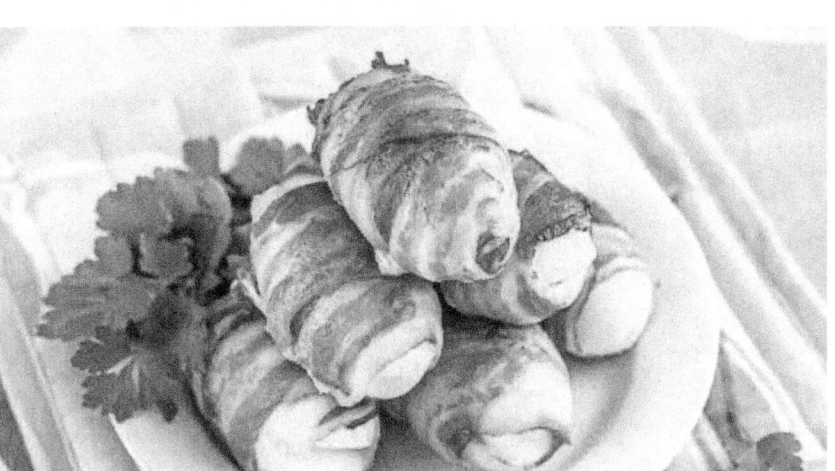

Eggs wrapped in crispy bacon and topped with soft cheese create a deliciously rich and savory breakfast treat. This dish is both satisfying and easy to make.

INGREDIENTS

- 4 large eggs
- 4 slices of bacon
- 2 oz soft cheese (e.g., cream cheese, brie)
- Salt, to taste
- Freshly ground black pepper (as much as preferred)

NUTRITIONAL INFO

Cal 380 • Fat 30 g • Carb 1 g • Protein 25 g

ALLERGEN INFO

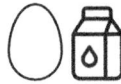

INSTRUCTIONS

1. Commence by preheating the oven to 400°F (200°C).
2. Grease a muffin tin or line it with parchment paper.
3. Wrap each slice of bacon around the sides of each muffin cup, creating a bacon cup.
4. Crack an egg into each bacon cup.
5. Season with salt and pepper.
6. Cook in the oven until the bacon turns crispy and the egg whites are cooked completely while keeping the yolks slightly runny, typically 15 to 18 minutes.
7. Remove from the oven and let cool for a few minutes.
8. Gently remove the bacon-wrapped eggs from the muffin tin.
9. Place a spoonful of soft cheese on each bacon-wrapped egg.

EGG MUFFINS

SERVING 2
PREP TIME: 5 MIN
COOK TIME: 20 MIN

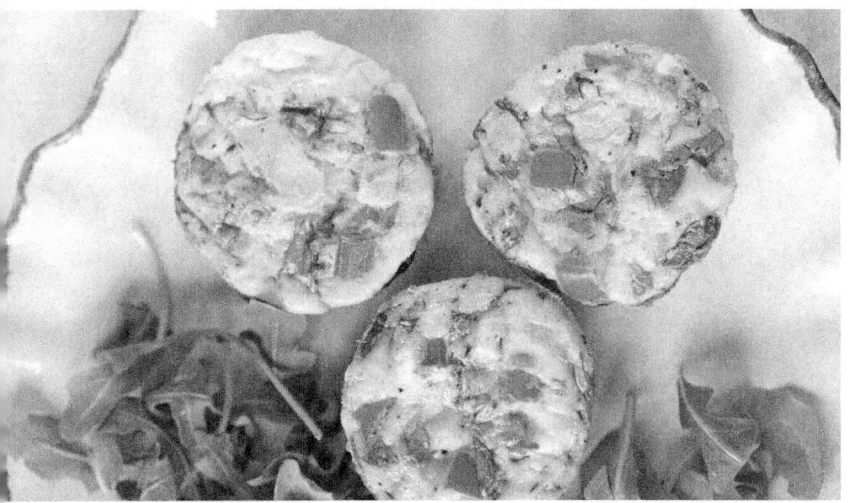

These portable egg muffins, packed with crumbled bacon, are perfect for a quick breakfast on the go. They are simple to prepare and can be customized with your favorite ingredients.

INGREDIENTS

- 6 large eggs
- 1/4 lb. cooked bacon, crumbled
- Salt, to taste
- Freshly ground black pepper (as much as preferred)
- Drizzle beef tallow

NUTRITIONAL INFO

Cal 280 • Fat 20 g • Carb 1 g • Protein 25 g

ALLERGEN INFO

INSTRUCTIONS

1. Commence by setting the oven's temperature to 375°F (190°C). Grease a muffin tin using olive oil or beef tallow.
2. In one bowl, beat the eggs together. Season with salt and pepper.
3. Divide the crumbled bacon evenly among the muffin cups.
4. Pour the beaten eggs over the bacon in each muffin cup, filling each about 3/4 full.
5. Bake in the oven until the egg muffins are set and slightly golden brown on top, about 20-25 minutes.
6. Remove from the oven and let cool for a few minutes before serving.
7. Optionally, garnish with chopped herbs or shredded cheese if desired.

BEEF OMELET

SERVING 2
PREP TIME: 5 MIN
COOK TIME: 10 MIN

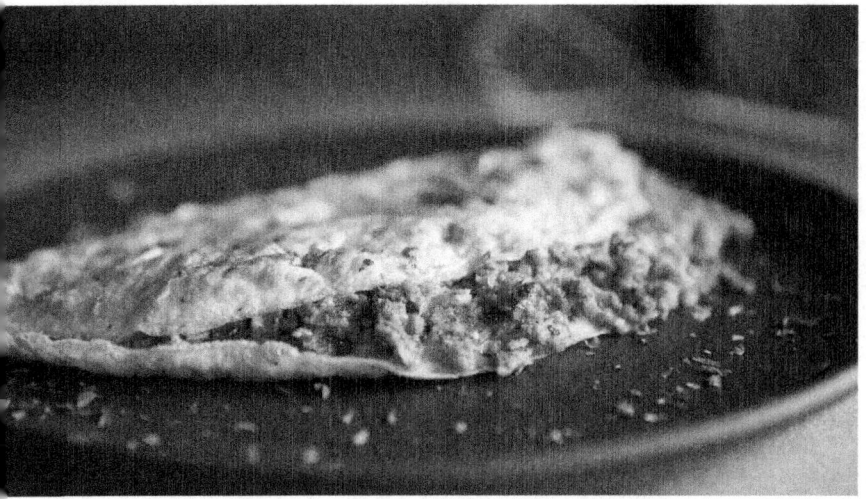

A flavorful omelet stuffed with ground beef provides a protein-rich meal to kickstart your morning. It's a fulfilling dish that combines the best of beef and eggs.

INGREDIENTS

- 4 large eggs
- 1/2 lb ground beef
- Salt, to taste
- Freshly ground black pepper (as much as preferred)
- Drizzle beef tallow

NUTRITIONAL INFO

Cal 350 • Fat 25 g • Carb 1 g • Protein 30 g

ALLERGEN INFO

INSTRUCTIONS

1. Heat a drizzle of olive oil or beef tallow in a skillet over medium heat.
2. Put the ground beef into the skillet, breaking it apart using a spatula. Fry until it is browned and cooked, which should take about 7 to 10 minutes.
3. Crack the eggs into a mixing bowl while the beef cooks. Gently whisk the ingredients using a fork, and then add salt or pepper to season the mixture.
4. After the beef has been cooked, you can move it to one side of the skillet and then pour the beaten eggs into the empty space.
5. Continue cooking the eggs without interruption for a minute or two until they begin to solidify around the edges.
6. When cooking eggs, you can gently use a spatula, pushing the cooked edges towards the center of the skillet while tilting it to let the uncooked eggs flow to the edges.
7. After the eggs have mostly set but are still slightly runny on top, you can spoon the cooked ground beef over one side of the omelet.
8. Carefully fold the other half of the omelet over the beef filling.
9. Cook for another minute to heat through and set the eggs.
10. Carefully transfer the cooked omelet onto a plate and serve it immediately while it's still hot.

SAUSAGE SCRAMBLE

SERVING 2
PREP TIME: 5 MIN
COOK TIME: 10 MIN

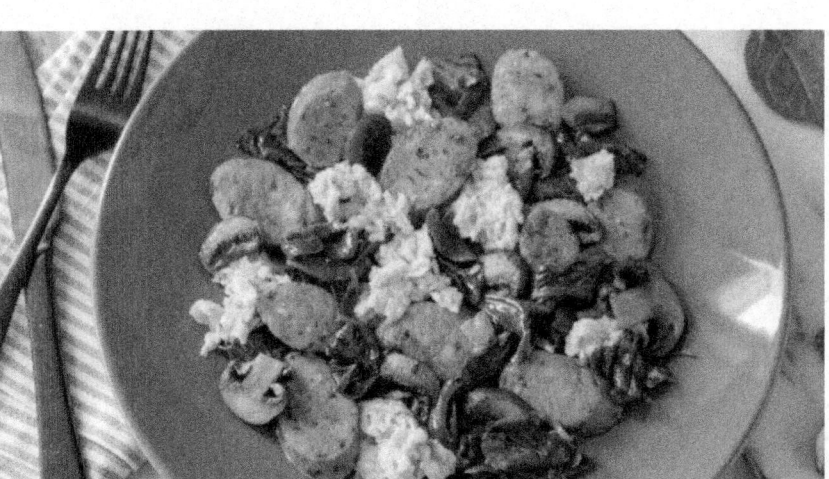

This savory scramble, made with breakfast sausage and eggs, is perfect for a hearty and quick breakfast. It's packed with flavor and easy to whip up any morning.

INGREDIENTS

- 6 large eggs
- 1/2 lb breakfast sausage
- Salt, to taste
- Freshly ground black pepper (as much as preferred)
- Drizzle beef tallow

NUTRITIONAL INFO

Cal 350 • Fat 25 g • Carb 1 g • Protein 30 g

ALLERGEN INFO

INSTRUCTIONS

1. Heat a drizzle of olive oil or beef tallow in a skillet over medium heat.
2. Be sure to take the sausage out of its casing and break it up as you put it into the skillet.
3. Fry the sausage until it is cooked and browned over medium heat, using a spatula to break it apart as it cooks. This process takes 7 to 10 minutes.
4. Crack the eggs into a mixing bowl while the sausage cooks. After whisking the eggs lightly with a fork, proceed to season with salt and pepper.
5. Once the sausage is cooked, pour the beaten eggs into the skillet with the sausage.
6. Stir continuously with a spatula, scrambling the eggs with the sausage, until the eggs are fully cooked and scrambled, about 3–5 minutes.

CARNIVORE BREAKFAST
PIZZA

SERVING 2
PREP TIME: 5 MIN
COOK TIME: 20 MIN

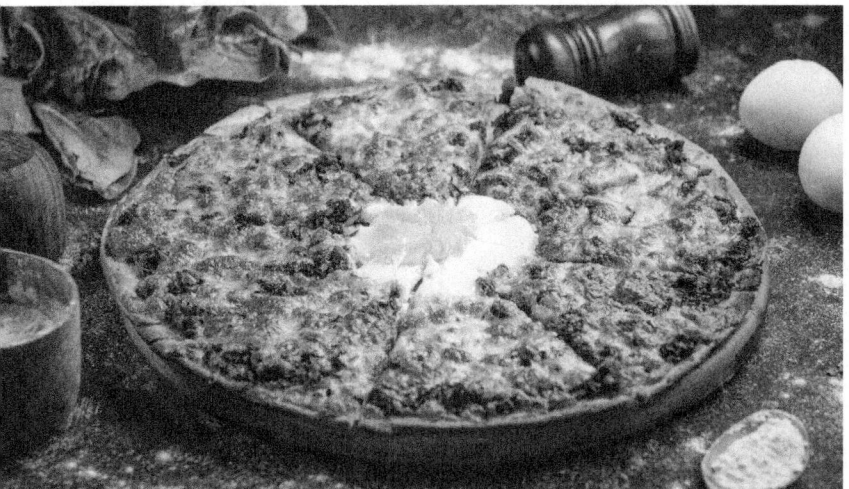

This breakfast pizza features a ground beef crust topped with eggs and optional cheese. It's a unique and satisfying way to enjoy a morning meal, a fun twist on traditional breakfast items.

INGREDIENTS

- 1/2 lb ground beef
- 4 large eggs
- 1/2 cup shredded cheese (optional)
- Salt, to taste (optional)
- Freshly ground black pepper (as much as preferred) (optional)
- 1 cup pork rinds, crushed

NUTRITIONAL INFO

Cal 400 • Fat 30 g • Carb 1 g • Protein 35 g

ALLERGEN INFO

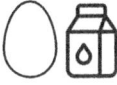

INSTRUCTIONS

1. Commence by preheating the oven to 400°F (200°C).
2. Fry the ground beef (over medium heat) in a skillet until browned and cooked, breaking it apart with a spatula, about 7–10 minutes.
3. Crack the eggs into a mixing bowl while the beef is cooking. Lightly mix the eggs with a fork and add pepper or salt to taste, if preferred.
4. Once the beef is cooked, spread it evenly on a baking sheet to form a "crust".
5. Pour the beaten eggs over the beef "crust", spreading them evenly.
6. Sprinkle shredded cheese over the eggs if using.
7. Bake in the oven for 10-15 minutes or until the eggs are set and the cheese is melted and bubbly.
8. Remove from the oven and sprinkle crushed pork rinds over the top.
9. Slice and serve hot.

CHEESE-CRUSTED HAM
AND EGG SANDWICH

SERVING 2
PREP TIME: 5 MIN
COOK TIME: 10 MIN

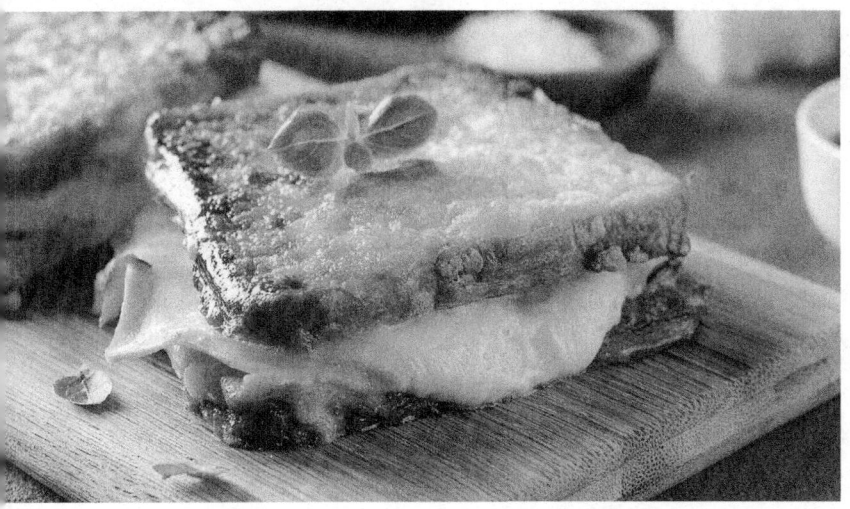

A delectable sandwich, it features eggs and ham enveloped in a crispy cheese crust. It's a delicious and filling way to start your day with a crunch.

INGREDIENTS

- 4 slices of ham
- 4 large eggs
- 1 cup shredded cheese

NUTRITIONAL INFO

Cal 380 • Fat 30 g • Carb 1 g • Protein 30 g

ALLERGEN INFO

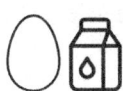

INSTRUCTIONS

1. Make sure to preheat the oven to 375°F (190°C).
2. Place the ham slices in pairs on a parchment paper-lined baking sheet, making sure they slightly overlap.
3. Crack an egg into the center of each pair of ham slices.
4. Sprinkle shredded cheese evenly over each egg.
5. Bake the dish in the oven after preheating until the egg whites are cooked completely and the cheese has melted and become bubbly, which typically takes about 8 to 10 minutes.
6. Take out the ham and egg sandwiches from the oven and gently place them onto a plate.
7. Optionally, garnish with chopped herbs or additional shredded cheese if desired.

CARNIVORE DIET
BREAKFAST TACOS

SERVING 2
PREP TIME: 5 MIN
COOK TIME: 10 MIN

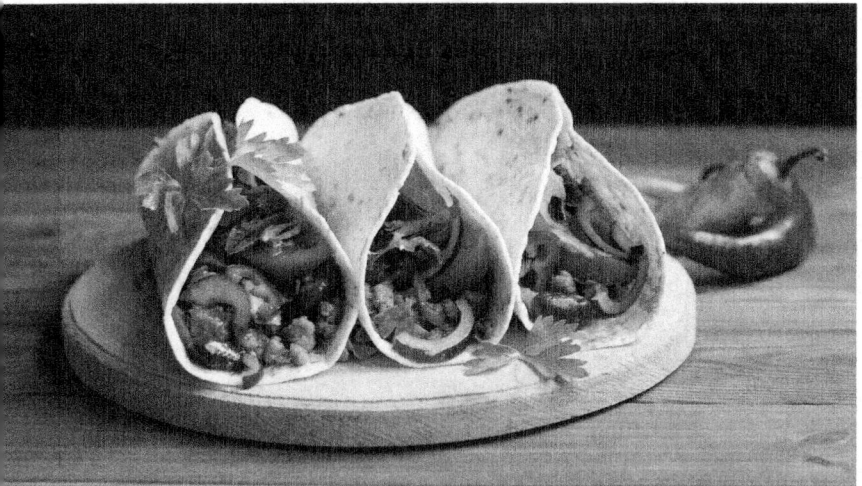

These breakfast tacos use bacon slices as the shell, filled with a savory mix of scrambled eggs and ground beef. It's a creative and protein-rich twist on traditional tacos.

INGREDIENTS

- 4 large eggs
- 1/2 lb ground beef
- 4 slices of bacon
- 1/2 cup shredded cheese (optional)
- Salt, to taste
- Freshly ground black pepper (as much as preferred)

NUTRITIONAL INFO

Cal 350 • Fat 25 g • Carb 0 g • Protein 30 g

ALLERGEN INFO

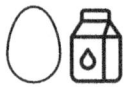

INSTRUCTIONS

1. Fry the bacon in a skillet (over medium heat) until it becomes crispy. Remove and set aside on a paper towel-lined plate.
2. Into the skillet add the ground beef and cook until it is browned and cooked, about 7-10 minutes. Remember to season with salt and pepper.
3. Whisk the eggs in a mixing bowl while the beef is cooking—season with salt and pepper.
4. Transfer the beaten eggs into the pan along with the cooked ground beef. Ensure to keep stirring until the eggs are completely cooked and have turned into scrambled eggs, which should take approximately 3 to 5 minutes.
5. Lay the cooked bacon slices on a plate and evenly distribute the beef and egg mixture over each slice.
6. Sprinkle shredded cheese over the beef and egg mixture if desired.
7. Optionally, roll the bacon slices around the filling to form taco-like wraps.

SNACKS, SIDES, AND SALADS

48 CHEESE CRISPY ROLL STUFFED WITH SOFT CHEESE
49 DEVILED EGGS
50 FRIED CHICKEN SKIN
51 CHEESE BALLS
52 BEEF BONE MARROW CUSTARD
53 CARNIVORE MAYONNAISE
54 TUNA AND EGG SALAD
55 DUCK LIVER MOUSSE
56 CARNIVORE DIET TURKEY BACON-WRAPPED MOZZARELLA STICKS
57 MEAT ASSORTED SALAD WITH BLUE CHEESE
58 MEAT BREAD
59 BEEF JERKY

CHEESE CRISPY ROLL
STUFFED WITH SOFT CHEESE

SERVING 2
PREP TIME: 5 MIN
COOK TIME: 10 MIN

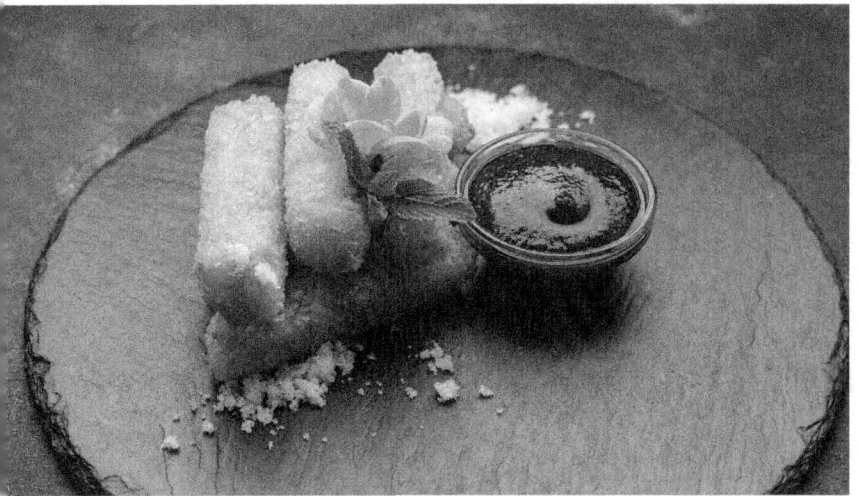

Delight in these crunchy cheese rolls filled with creamy soft cheese. They're perfect as a snack or a savory appetizer.

INGREDIENTS

- 1 cup shredded cheese (cheddar, parmesan, or your choice)
- 4 tablespoons soft cheese (cream cheese, brie, or your choice)

NUTRITIONAL INFO

Cal 300 • Fat 25 g • Carb 1 g • Protein 15 g

ALLERGEN INFO

INSTRUCTIONS

1. Commence by setting the oven's temperature to 375°F (190°C).
2. Cover the baking sheet with parchment paper.
3. Place small mounds (about 2 tablespoons each) of shredded cheese onto the parchment paper, spacing them about 2 inches apart.
4. Flatten each small mound using the back of a spoon to create small circles.
5. Put in the oven until the cheese has melted and the edges have turned a golden brown color, for approximately 5 to 7 minutes.
6. Remove from the oven and let the cheese circles cool for about 1 minute to firm up slightly but remain pliable.
7. Place a tablespoon of soft cheese in the center of each cheese circle.
8. Carefully roll the cheese circle around the soft cheese to form a roll.
9. Let the rolls cool and firm on the baking sheet for a few more minutes before serving.

DEVILED EGGS

SERVING 2
PREP TIME: 5 MIN
COOK TIME: 15 MIN

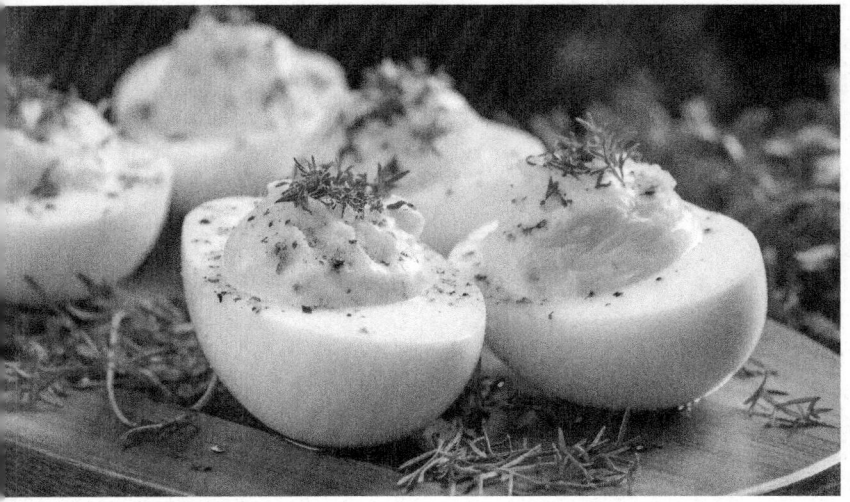

Classic deviled eggs with a carnivore twist, featuring a rich and creamy filling, are ideal for a tasty snack or a light side dish.

INGREDIENTS

- 4 large eggs
- 2 tablespoons mayonnaise (carnivore-friendly)
- Salt, to taste
- Freshly ground black pepper (as much as preferred)

NUTRITIONAL INFO

Cal 250 • Fat 20 g • Carb 1 g • Protein 12 g

ALLERGEN INFO

INSTRUCTIONS

1. Place the eggs in a saucepan and cover them with water. Bring to a boil over medium-high heat.
2. After the water comes to a rolling boil, cover the saucepan after taking it off the heat, leaving the eggs for 10-12 minutes.
3. Pour out the hot water and then place the eggs into a bowl of ice water to cool for a few minutes.
4. Peel the eggs and slice them in half lengthwise.
5. Remove the yolks and place them in a small mixing bowl.
6. Using a fork, crush the egg yolks and then combine them with mayonnaise, salt, and pepper until the mixture becomes smooth.
7. Place the yolk mixture into the egg white halves using a spoon.
8. Serve right away, or keep it in the refrigerator until you're ready to enjoy it.

FRIED CHICKEN SKIN

SERVING 2
PREP TIME: 5 MIN
COOK TIME: 5 MIN

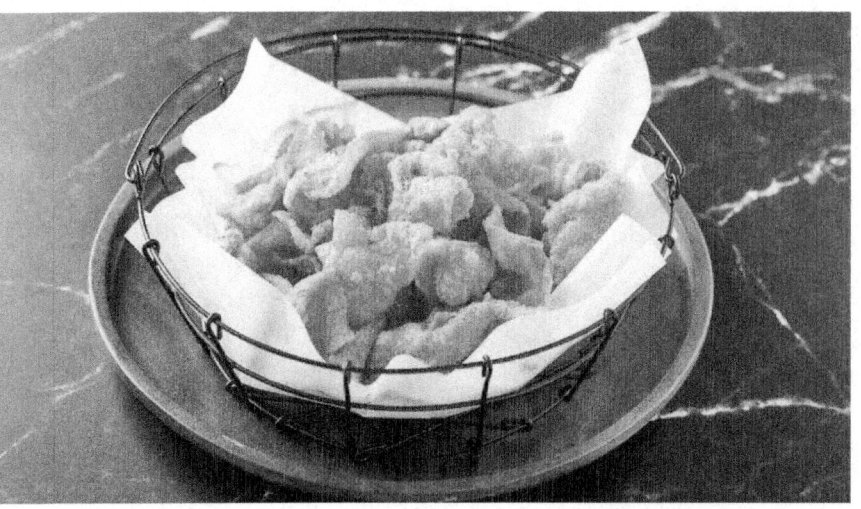

Crispy fried chicken skin seasoned to perfection. It's a crunchy, flavorful snack that's hard to resist.

INGREDIENTS

- 1 lb chicken skin
- Salt, to taste
- Freshly ground black pepper (as much as preferred)
- Drizzle of beef tallow or other animal fat for frying

NUTRITIONAL INFO

Cal 300 • Fat 20 g • Carb 1 g • Protein 30 g

INSTRUCTIONS

1. When cooking, warm up a small quantity of beef tallow or another type of animal fat in a skillet over medium heat.
2. Season the chicken skin by sprinkling salt and pepper on it.
3. Add the chicken skin in a single layer once the skillet is hot.
4. Fry the chicken skin until golden brown and crispy, about 3-5 minutes per side.
5. Take out the fried chicken skin and drain it on paper towels, then remove excess fat.
6. Let it cool for a minute or two before serving.

CHEESE BALLS

SERVING 2
PREP TIME: 5 MIN
COOK TIME: 30 MIN

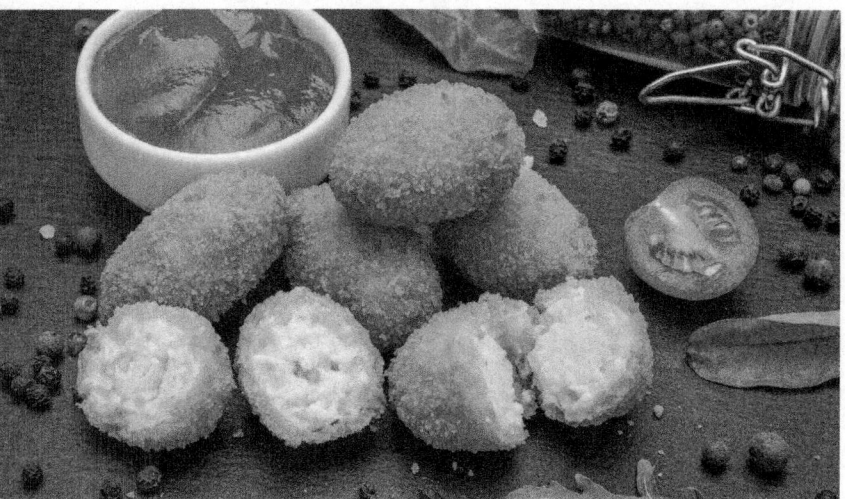

These savory cheese balls are packed with rich, cheesy goodness. They're great for a quick snack or as a party appetizer.

INGREDIENTS

- 1 cup shredded cheese (cheddar, gouda, or your choice)
- 2 oz cream cheese, softened
- Salt, to taste (optional)
- Freshly ground black pepper (as much as preferred) (optional)
- Optional coating: crushed pork rinds, chopped bacon bits

INSTRUCTIONS

1. Mix the shredded cheese and softened cream cheese in a mixing bowl. Mix well until thoroughly combined.
2. If you'd like, you can add salt and pepper to the mixture to season it to your liking.
3. Divide the cheese mixture into 2 equal portions.
4. Roll each part into a ball by shaping it with your hands.
5. Roll the cheese balls in crushed pork rinds or chopped bacon bits for an additional crunchy coating.
6. Place the cheese balls on a plate or baking sheet lined with parchment paper.
7. To achieve a firmer texture, it's best to put the cheese balls into the refrigerator for at least 30 minutes.
8. Serve chilled as a snack or appetizer.

NUTRITIONAL INFO

Cal 400 • Fat 35 g • Carb 2 g • Protein 20 g

ALLERGEN INFO

BEEF BONE MARROW CUSTARD

SERVING 2
PREP TIME: 5 MIN
COOK TIME: 25 MIN

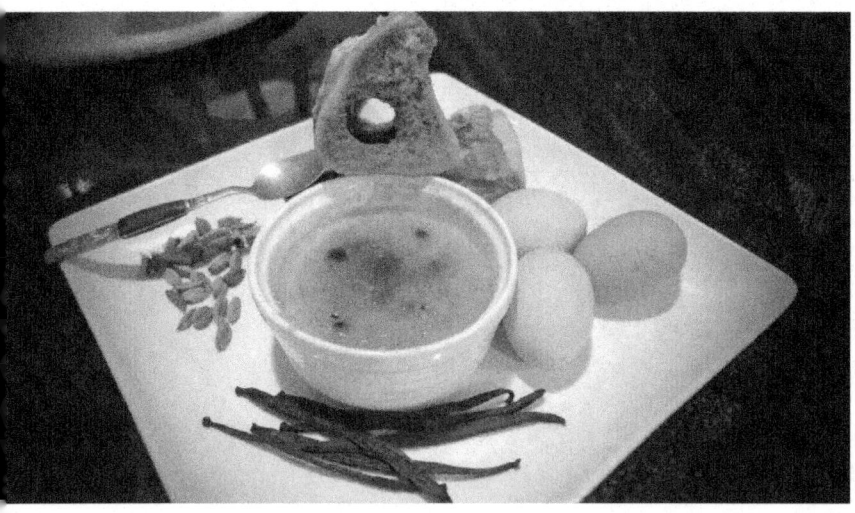

A luxurious custard made with rich beef bone marrow. A decadent treat for special occasions.

INGREDIENTS

- 1/2 lb beef bone marrow
- 2 large eggs
- 1/4 cup heavy cream
- Salt, to taste
- Freshly ground black pepper (as much as preferred)
- Optional: chopped herbs for garnish

NUTRITIONAL INFO

Cal 400 • Fat 40 g • Carb 1 g • Protein 10 g

ALLERGEN INFO

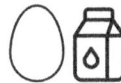

INSTRUCTIONS

1. Make certain to preheat the oven to 350°F (175°C).
2. Place the beef bone marrow in an oven-safe dish and roast in the oven until the marrow is soft and quickly scooped out about 20-25 minutes.
3. In the meantime, in a mixing bowl, vigorously mix the eggs and heavy cream until they are thoroughly combined.
4. Add salt to the egg mixture and a grind of black pepper until it suits your taste.
5. Once the bone marrow is done, remove it from the oven and cool slightly.
6. Scoop out the softened bone marrow and add it to the egg mixture. Mix well.
7. Pour the mixture into two ramekins or small oven-safe dishes.
8. Place the ramekins in a baking dish and fill the dish with hot water to create a water bath around the ramekins.
9. Bake in the oven that has been preheated until the custard is firm and slightly golden on top, typically for 15 to 20 minutes.
10. After baking, take the custards out of the oven and let them cool for a few minutes before serving.

CARNIVORE MAYONNAISE

SERVING 2
PREP TIME: 5 MIN
COOK TIME: 20 MIN

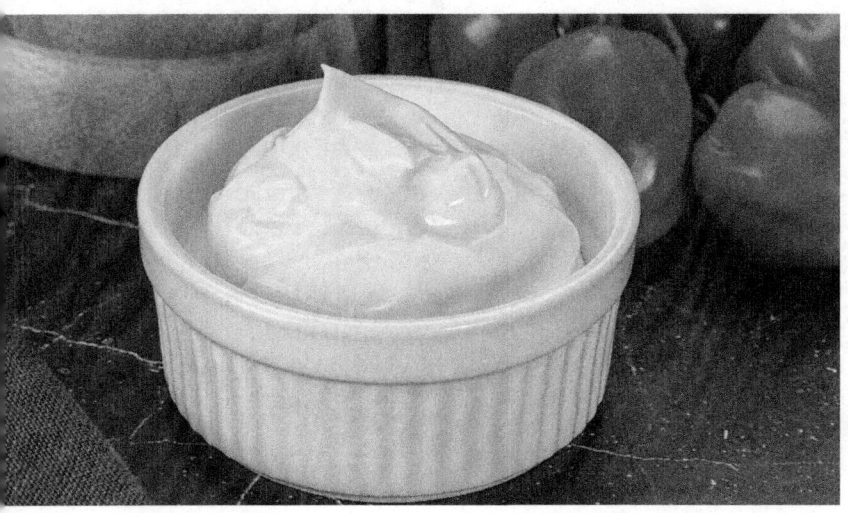

A rich and creamy homemade mayonnaise perfect for enhancing any carnivore dish. Easy to make and deliciously satisfying.

INGREDIENTS

- 2 large egg yolks
- 1 cup beef tallow, melted and cooled slightly
- 1 tablespoon lemon juice
- Salt, to taste

NUTRITIONAL INFO

Cal 100 • Fat 12 g • Carb 0 g • Protein 5 g

ALLERGEN INFO

INSTRUCTIONS

1. Mix the egg yolks and lemon juice using a blender or food processor until they are thoroughly combined.
2. While the blender is running, start adding the melted beef tallow in a steady stream until the mixture is emulsified and thickened.
3. Blend for another 30 seconds to ensure everything is well combined.
4. Add salt to the mixture to your preference and blend it briefly once more to ensure the salt is fully incorporated.
5. Place the carnivore mayonnaise in a jar or airtight container and keep it in the refrigerator until you are ready to use it.

TUNA AND EGG SALAD

SERVING 2
PREP TIME: 5 MIN
COOK TIME: 15 MIN

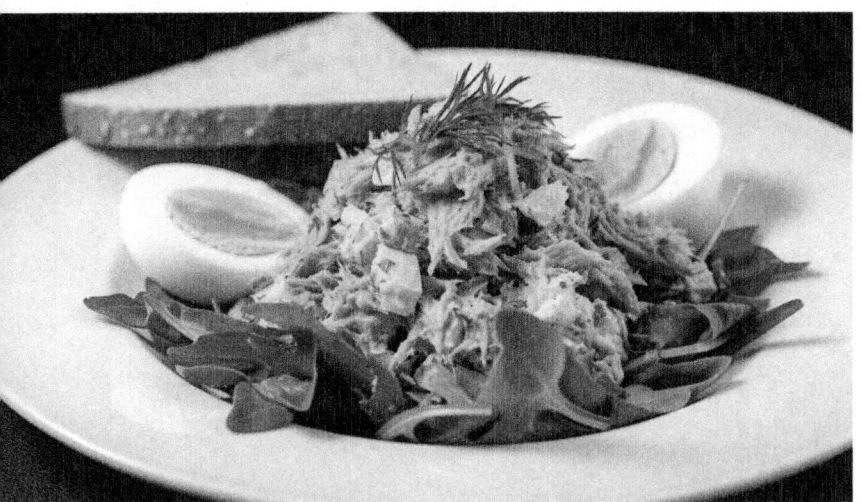

A hearty salad combining tender tuna and diced eggs, bound with carnivore mayonnaise. Great for a protein-packed meal.

INGREDIENTS

- 2 cans (5 oz each) of drained tuna
- 2 tablespoons carnivore mayonnaise
- 3 large eggs, hard-boiled and diced
- Salt, to taste
- Freshly ground black pepper (as much as preferred)

INSTRUCTIONS

1. Combine the drained tuna, diced hard-boiled eggs, and carnivore mayonnaise in a mixing bowl.
2. Season with salt and pepper to taste.
3. Combine all ingredients thoroughly until they are evenly coated with the mayonnaise.

NUTRITIONAL INFO

Cal 500 • Fat 32 g • Carb 1 g • Protein 53 g

ALLERGEN INFO

DUCK LIVER MOUSSE

SERVING 2
PREP TIME: 5 MIN
COOK TIME: 10 MIN

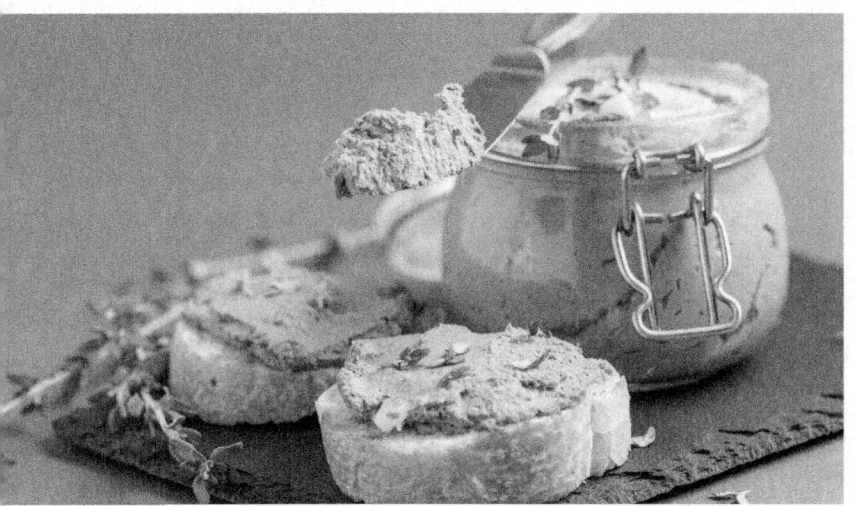

Smooth and creamy duck liver mousse, rich in flavor, and perfect as a gourmet snack. Serve with carnivore-friendly accompaniments.

INGREDIENTS

- 1 lb duck liver
- 1/2 cup rendered duck fat
- Salt to taste
- Optional: herbs and spices of your choice

NUTRITIONAL INFO

Cal 300 • Fat 15 g • Carb 0g • Protein 25 g

INSTRUCTIONS

1. Rinse the duck liver under cold water and pat dry with paper towels.
2. Make the rendered duck fat melt in a skillet until it is hot but not smoking.
3. Add the duck liver to the skillet until it is browned on all sides and cooked through, about 3-5 minutes per side.
4. Transfer the duck liver to a food processor or blender once cooked.
5. Add the rendered duck fat to the food processor or blender with the duck liver.
6. Blend the duck liver and fat together until the mixture is smooth and creamy, making sure to scrape down the sides of the bowl as necessary.
7. Season the duck liver mousse with salt to taste and, optionally, any herbs and spices you desire.
8. Transfer the duck liver mousse to a serving dish or storage container.

CARNIVORE DIET TURKEY BACON-
WRAPPED MOZZARELLA STICKS

SERVING 2
PREP TIME: 10 MIN
COOK TIME: 15 MIN

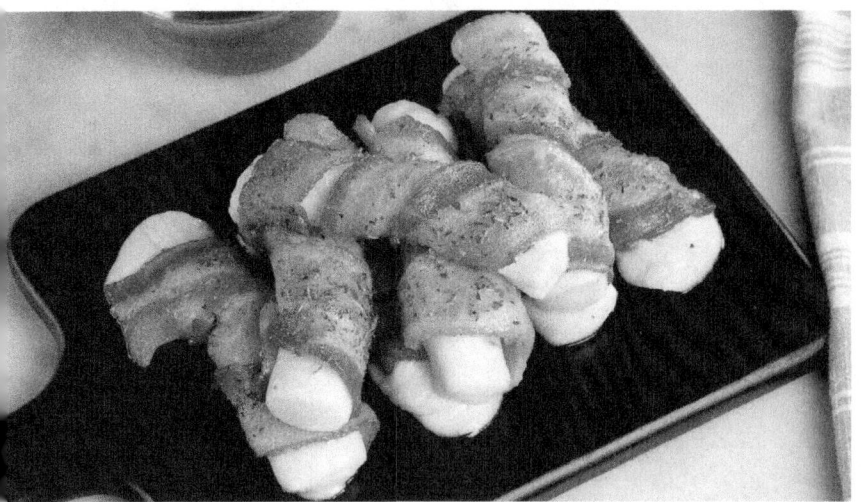

Gooey mozzarella sticks wrapped in crispy turkey bacon. An indulgent snack that's easy to prepare and enjoy.

INGREDIENTS

- 6 mozzarella cheese sticks
- 12 slices of turkey bacon

NUTRITIONAL INFO

Cal 200 • Fat 15 g • Carb 2g • Protein 25 g

ALLERGEN INFO

INSTRUCTIONS

1. Commence by preheating your oven to 400°F (200°C).
2. Cut each mozzarella cheese stick in half to make 12 shorter sticks.
3. Wrap each mozzarella stick with a slice of turkey bacon, covering the entire cheese stick.
4. Arrange the bacon-wrapped mozzarella sticks on a baking tray.
5. Place the dish in the oven and cook for 12-15 minutes or until the turkey bacon reaches a crispy texture and the cheese is fully melted.

MEAT ASSORTED SALAD
WITH BLUE CHEESE

SERVING 2
PREP TIME: 15 MIN
COOK TIME: 15 MIN

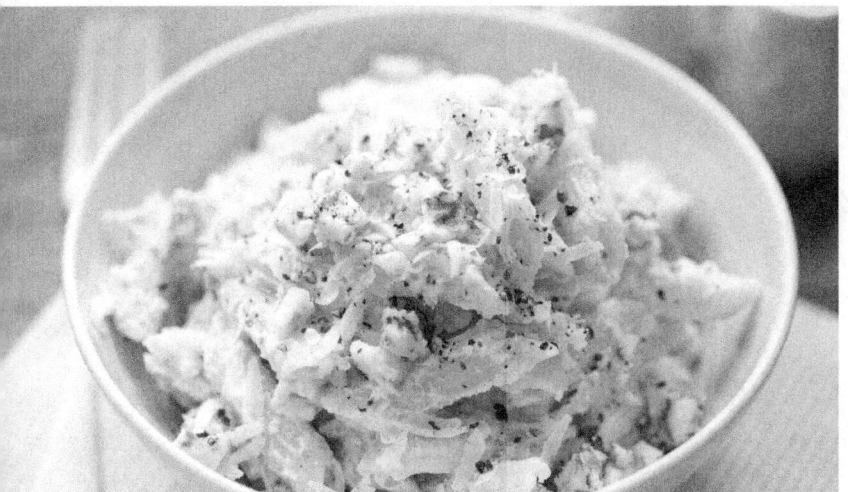

A robust salad featuring a mix of meats and crumbled blue cheese. Perfect for a satisfying and flavorful side dish.

INGREDIENTS

- 1 cup cooked chicken, shredded or diced
- 1 cup cooked beef, shredded or diced
- 2 hard-boiled eggs, diced
- 2 tablespoons carnivore mayonnaise
- 1/4 cup crumbled blue cheese

INSTRUCTIONS

1. Combine the cooked chicken, cooked beef, and diced hard-boiled eggs in a large mixing bowl.
2. Add the carnivore mayonnaise and mix until everything is evenly coated.
3. Gently fold in the crumbled blue cheese.
4. If preferred, season with salt and pepper to taste.
5. Serve right away or store in the refrigerator until you're ready to serve.

NUTRITIONAL INFO

Cal 600 • Fat 45 g • Carb 2g • Protein 50 g

ALLERGEN INFO

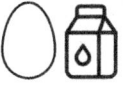

MEAT BREAD

SERVING 2
PREP TIME: 15 MIN
COOK TIME: 30 MIN

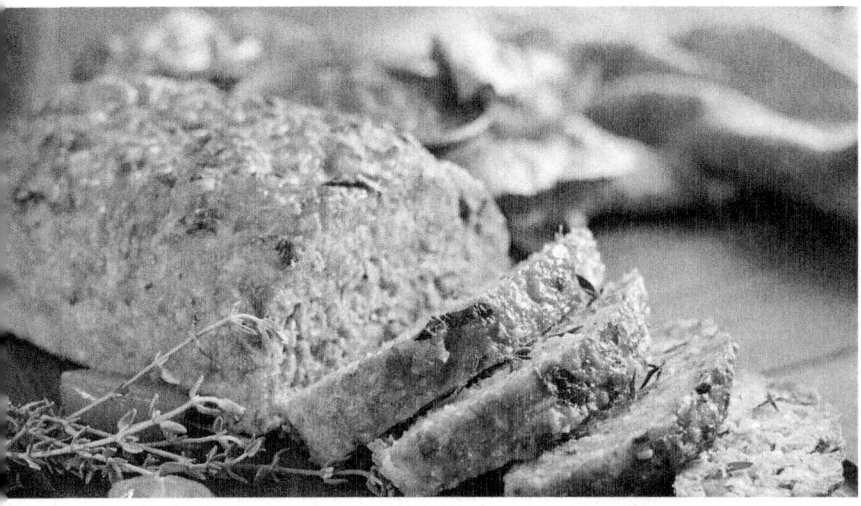

This hearty meat bread is made with ground meat and eggs, offering a protein-rich alternative to traditional bread. Great as a snack or side dish.

INGREDIENTS

- 1 lb ground beef (also can use chicken, turkey, or pork)
- 2 large eggs
- 1/2 cup grated cheese (optional)
- Salt, to taste
- Freshly ground black pepper (as much as preferred)

NUTRITIONAL INFO

Cal 450 • Fat 30 g • Carb 1g • Protein 40 g

ALLERGEN INFO

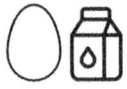

INSTRUCTIONS

1. Make sure to preheat the oven to 375°F (190°C).
2. In a bowl (large enough), mix the eggs, ground beef, grated cheese (if using), salt, and pepper. Thoroughly combine all ingredients by mixing well until fully incorporated.
3. Transfer the meat mixture into a loaf pan and firmly press it down to ensure it holds together.
4. Place in the oven and bake until the meat is cooked (30-35 minutes) and the top has turned golden brown.
5. Take the dish out of the oven and let it cool for a few minutes before slicing it and serving.

BEEF JERKY

SERVING 2
PREP TIME: 15 MIN
COOK TIME: 4-6 HOURS

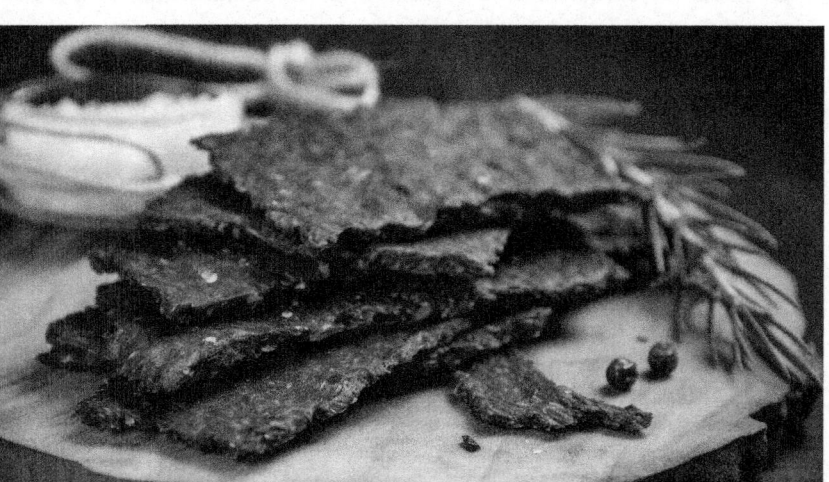

Homemade beef jerky, seasoned and dried to perfection. It is a convenient and high-protein snack for any time of the day.

INGREDIENTS

- 1 lb beef (top round, flank steak, or sirloin)
- 1 teaspoon salt
- 1 teaspoon black pepper
- 1 teaspoon garlic powder (optional)
- 1 teaspoon onion powder (optional)

NUTRITIONAL INFO

Cal 250 • Fat 10 g • Carb 0g • Protein 40 g

INSTRUCTIONS

1. Place the beef in the freezer for 1-2 hours to firm it up and make it easier to slice.
2. When preparing beef jerky, it is important to slice the beef into thin strips. If you cut against the grain, it will result in a more tender jerky, while cutting with the grain will give a chewier texture.
3. Combine the garlic powder, salt, onion powder, and black pepper in a large mixing bowl.
4. Place the beef strips into the bowl and toss them to ensure an even coating with the seasoning.
5. Place the seasoned beef strips in a resealable plastic bag or a covered container.
6. Chill for at least 4 hours, or preferably overnight, to ensure the flavors permeate the meat.
7. Commence by preheating your oven to 175°F (80°C) or setting a dehydrator to the meat setting.
8. Make sure the beef strips are arranged in a single layer on a wire rack (set it over a baking sheet) or on the trays of the dehydrator.
9. Dry the beef in the oven or dehydrator for 4-6 hours or until the jerky is dry but still slightly pliable.
10. Allow the beef jerky to cool completely before storing it in an airtight container.
11. Store at room temperature for up to a week or refrigerate for a longer shelf life.

BEEF

61 GRILLED BEEF KABOBS WITH GARLIC HERB BUTTER
62 BEEF CHUCK ROAST WITH ROSEMARY AU JUS
63 BEEF BACON-WRAPPED MEATLOAF
64 COFFEE-RUBBED BEEF BRISKET
65 GRILLED PORTERHOUSE STEAK
66 SMOKY BEEF TARTARE
67 BACON-WRAPPED FILET MIGNONS
68 FILET MIGNON WITH TRUFFLE BUTTER
69 RIBEYE STEAK WITH BLUE CHEESE BUTTER
70 BEEF TENDERLOIN MEDALLIONS WITH PEPPERCORN SAUCE
71 BEEF HEART STEAKS
72 BAKED BEEF CHOPS WITH MAYONNAISE AND CHEESE

GRILLED BEEF KABOBS
WITH GARLIC HERB BUTTER

SERVING 2
PREP TIME: 45 MIN
COOK TIME: 15 MIN

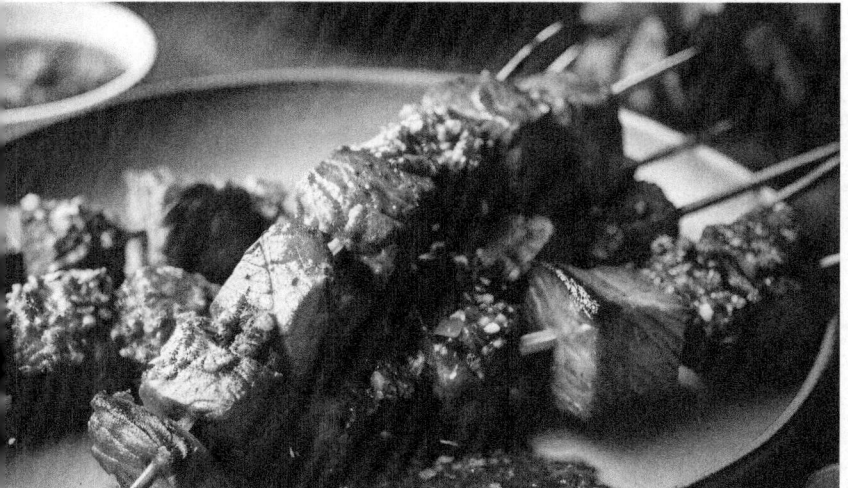

Succulent beef cubes grilled to perfection and basted with a rich garlic herb butter. These kabobs are a flavorful and satisfying option for any carnivore meal.

INGREDIENTS

- 1 lb beef cubes (such as sirloin or ribeye)
- 1/4 cup or 1/2 stick melted unsalted butter
- 2 minced garlic cloves
- 1 tablespoon chopped fresh herbs like rosemary, thyme, or parsley
- Salt and black pepper to taste
- Skewers, soaked in water if wooden

NUTRITIONAL INFO

Cal 450 • Fat 35 g • Carb 0 g • Protein 35 g

ALLERGEN INFO

INSTRUCTIONS

1. In a small bowl, blend the melted butter with minced garlic, chopped fresh herbs, black pepper, and salt. Thoroughly mix to prepare the garlic herb butter.
2. Arrange the beef cubes in a dish meant for lamb or swine.
3. Cover the beef cubes with half of the garlic herb butter, saving the remaining butter for basting.
4. Toss the meat cubes in the garlic-herb butter to ensure a uniform coating.
5. Cover the turkey or dish and let the beef cubes marinate in the refrigerator for thirty to sixty minutes.
6. Turn the heat up to medium-high on your grill.
7. Thread the marinated beef cubes onto the skewers, making sure to leave a tiny space between them.
8. Toss away any extra marinade.
9. Arrange the beef kabobs on the hot grill and cook for ten to fifteen minutes, rotating them once in between or until the beef is cooked to your preferred doneness and has a good sear on the outside.
10. Use a brush to brush the meat kabobs with the saved garlic herb butter while they are grilling.
11. Take the cooked beef kabobs off the grill and place them on a dish for serving.
12. Give the beef kabobs a few minutes to settle before presenting them.

BEEF CHUCK ROAST
WITH ROSEMARY AU JUS

SERVING 2
PREP TIME: 10 MIN
COOK TIME: 4-6 HOURS

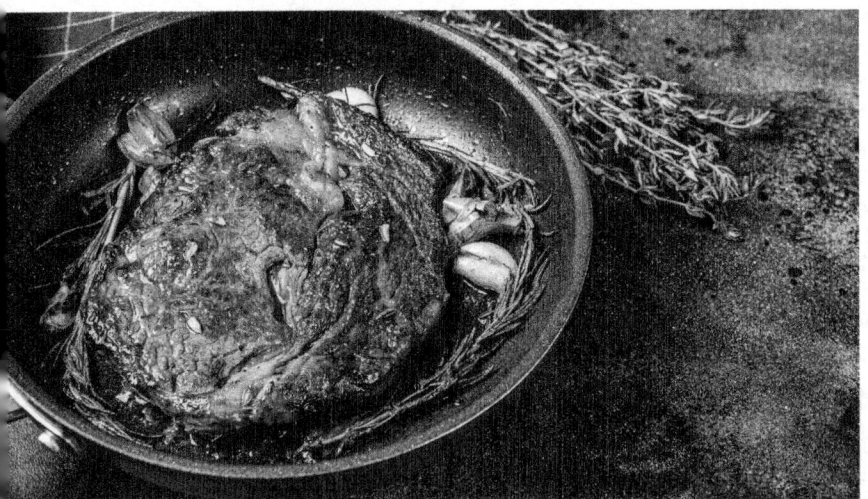

Tender beef chuck roast simmered with aromatic rosemary and served with a rich au jus is perfect for a hearty and comforting meal.

INGREDIENTS

- 1 to 1.5 lbs beef chuck roast
- 1 tablespoon fresh rosemary leaves, chopped
- 1 cup beef broth
- Salt and black pepper to taste

NUTRITIONAL INFO

Cal 450 • Fat 35 g • Carb 0 g • Protein 35 g

INSTRUCTIONS

1. Commence by preheating your oven to 325°F (160°C).
2. Liberally season the beef roast with salt and black pepper.
3. Drizzle the chopped rosemary over the roast beef.
4. Transfer the seared beef chuck roast to a little roasting pan or ovenproof plate.
5. Empty the beef brats into the pan, covering the bottom but exposing the roast.
6. Use a lid or aluminum foil to cover the pan.
7. Place the pan in the oven and let it roast for four to six hours, or until the beef roast reaches the desired tenderness and can be easily shredded.
8. After cooking, remove the roast beef from the oven and place it on a chopping board.
9. Give the beef roast a few minutes to rest before slicing or shredding.
10. Present the beef chuck roast slices or shredded meat with the pan-cooked rosemary au poivre.

BEEF BACON-WRAPPED
MEATLOAF

> **SERVING 2**
> PREP TIME: 10 MIN
> COOK TIME: 30 MIN

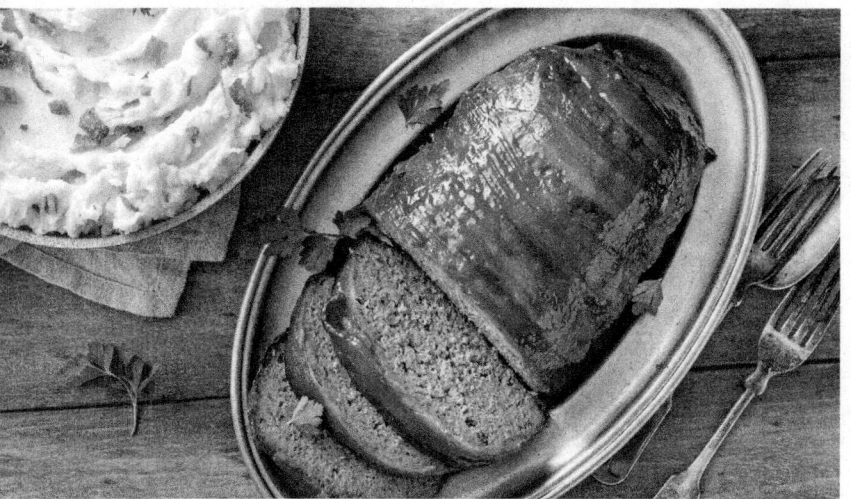

This meatloaf combines ground beef and crispy bacon, creating a juicy, flavorful dish. It's an excellent choice for a protein-packed dinner.

INGREDIENTS

- 1/2 lb ground beef
- 3-4 slices of beef bacon
- 1 egg
- Salt and black pepper to taste

NUTRITIONAL INFO

Cal 400 • Fat 25 g • Carb 0 g • Protein 30 g

ALLERGEN INFO

INSTRUCTIONS

1. Commence by preheating your oven to 375°F (190°C).
2. Combine the ground beef, egg, salt, and black pepper in a mixing bowl. Blend until thoroughly mixed.
3. Form the ground beef mixture into a small loaf, large enough to serve two people.
4. To ensure they cover the entire surface, wrap the beef bacon slices around the meatloaf.
5. Optional: You can weave the bacon slices for a decorative look if you'd like.
6. Transfer the meatloaf wrapped in bacon to a baking dish or sheet.
7. Bake the meatloaf in a preheated oven for 30 to 35 minutes or until the bacon is crispy and the meatloaf is fully cooked.
8. Once the meatloaf is done cooking, take it out of the oven and allow it to rest for a few minutes before you start slicing it.

COFFEE-RUBBED BEEF
BRISKET

SERVING 2
PREP TIME: 10 MIN
COOK TIME: 4-6 HOURS

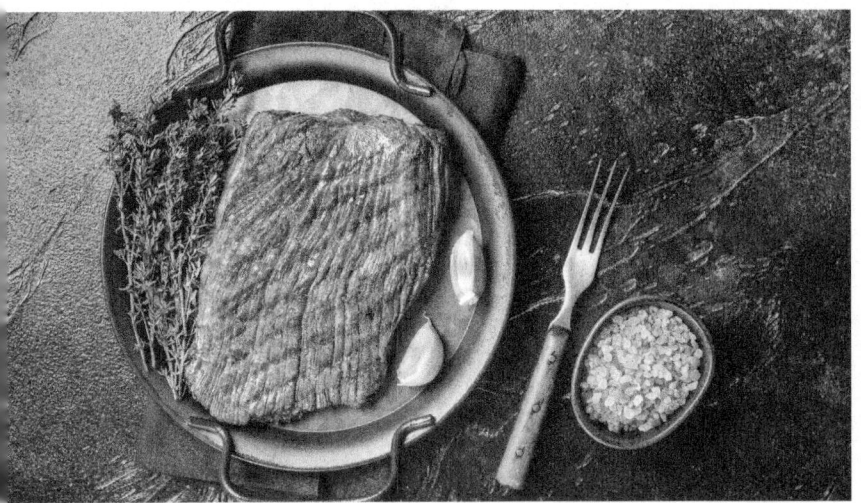

This unique brisket is rubbed with dark coffee grounds, offering a deep, smoky flavor. Slow-cooked to tender perfection, it is a showstopper.

INGREDIENTS

- 1 lb beef brisket
- 2 tablespoons coffee grounds (preferably dark roast)
- 1 tablespoon salt
- 1 tablespoon black pepper

NUTRITIONAL INFO

Cal 400 • Fat 30 g • Carb 1 g • Protein 30 g

INSTRUCTIONS

1. Commence by preheating your oven to 300°F (150°C).
2. Mix the coffee grounds, salt, and black pepper in a small bowl.
3. Pat the beef brisket dry with paper towels.
4. Rub the coffee mixture evenly over the surface of the brisket.
5. Place the brisket in a roasting pan or on an aluminum foil-lined baking sheet.
6. Cover the brisket loosely with foil.
7. Cook the brisket in the oven at the preheated temperature for 4-6 hours, or until it is tender enough and could be shredded with a fork.
8. When cooked, take the brisket out of the oven and let it rest for 10-15 minutes before slicing.
9. Slice the brisket against the grain into thin slices.

GRILLED PORTERHOUSE
STEAK

> **SERVING 2**
> PREP TIME: 10 MIN
> COOK TIME: 15 MIN

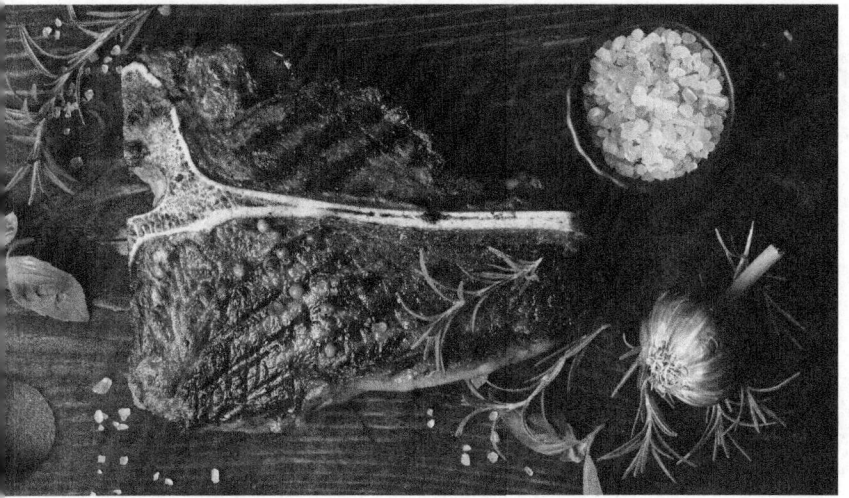

A juicy porterhouse steak seasoned simply with salt and pepper, then grilled to your desired doneness. This classic steakhouse favorite is sure to impress.

INGREDIENTS

- 1 porterhouse steak, about 1.5 lbs (approximately 1-inch thick)
- Salt and black pepper to taste
- Beef tallow for brushing

NUTRITIONAL INFO

Cal 600 • Fat 40 g • Carb 0 g • Protein 65 g

INSTRUCTIONS

1. Preheat your grill to high heat.
2. Remove the porterhouse steak from the refrigerator and let it sit at room temperature for 30 minutes to an hour before grilling. This helps ensure even cooking.
3. Make sure to pat the steak dry and remove any excess moisture.
4. Season both sides of the porterhouse steak generously with salt and black pepper.
5. Brush the grill grates (use olive oil or beef tallow) to prevent sticking.
6. Place the porterhouse steak on the hot grill and cook for about 5-7 minutes on each side for medium-rare or until the desired level of doneness is reached. Check for an internal temperature (use meat thermometer) of 130-135°F (54-57°C) for medium-rare, 140-145°F (60-63°C) for medium, or 150-155°F (65-68°C) for medium-well.
7. Remove the porterhouse steak from the grill once cooked to your liking and transfer it to a cutting board. Let it rest (5-10 minutes), allowing the juices to redistribute.
8. Slice the porterhouse steak against the grain into thick slices.

SMOKY BEEF TARTARE

SERVING 2
PREP TIME: 10 MIN
COOK TIME: 0 MIN

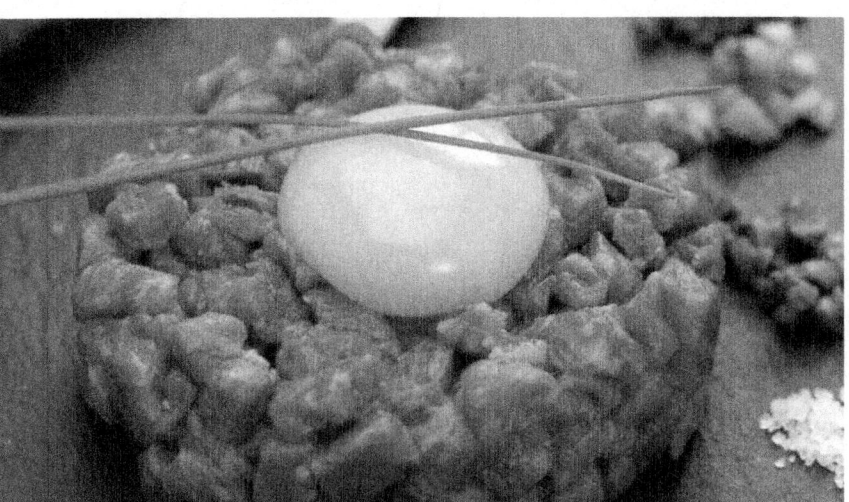

High-quality beef tenderloin is finely chopped and mixed with smoked beef tallow, creating a rich and flavorful tartare. This dish, served with a raw egg yolk, is for the adventurous palate.

INGREDIENTS

- 1/2 lb high-quality beef tenderloin or sirloin, finely chopped
- 2 large egg yolks
- 1 tablespoon smoked beef tallow or bacon fat
- 1 teaspoon smoked salt
- 1 teaspoon freshly ground black pepper
- 1 teaspoon mustard powder (optional, for slight tang)
- 1/2 teaspoon smoked paprika (optional for extra smokiness)

NUTRITIONAL INFO

Cal 300 • Fat 22 g • Carb 0 g • Protein 25 g

ALLERGEN INFO

INSTRUCTIONS

1. Ensure the beef is very cold before starting. Finely chop the beef tenderloin or sirloin by hand, aiming for a texture that is not too fine but not chunky.
2. Combine the finely chopped beef with the smoked beef tallow or bacon fat in a mixing bowl.
3. Add the smoked salt, freshly ground black pepper, and smoked paprika if using. Mix well.
4. If desired, mix in the mustard powder for an additional layer of flavor.
5. Divide the beef mixture into two equal portions and shape each into a neat mound or patty on individual plates.
6. Make a slight indentation on top of each mound and place a raw egg yolk in each indentation.
7. Serve the beef tartare immediately, garnished with additional smoked salt and black pepper if desired.

BACON-WRAPPED FILET
MIGNONS

SERVING 2
PREP TIME: 10 MIN
COOK TIME: 15 MIN

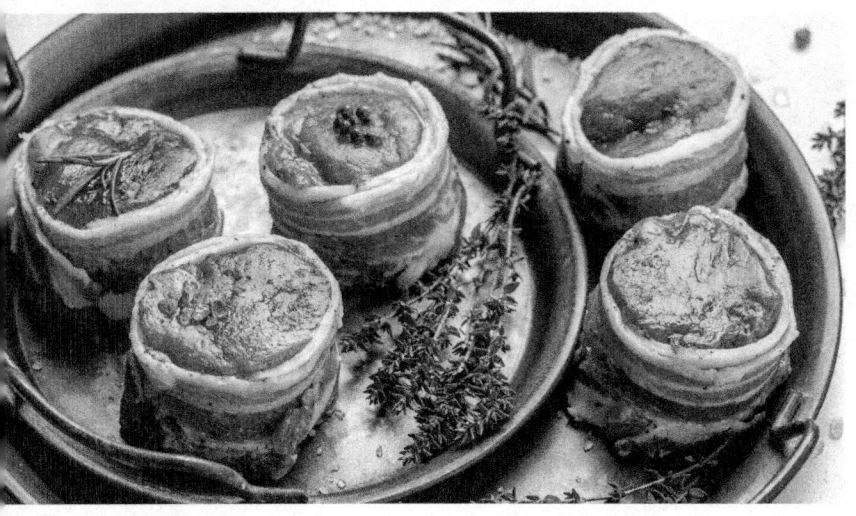

Tender filet mignon steaks wrapped in crispy bacon offer a luxurious and mouthwatering meal. An ideal choice for memorable events or an exquisite dining experience.

INGREDIENTS

- 2 filet mignon steaks, about 6 ounces each
- 4 slices of bacon
- Salt and black pepper to taste

NUTRITIONAL INFO

Cal 400 • Fat 30 g • Carb 0 g • Protein 30 g

INSTRUCTIONS

1. Commence by preheating your oven to 400°F (200°C).
2. Season the filet mignon steaks to taste with salt and black pepper.
3. Make sure the bacon completely encases the steak using two bacon pieces per filet mignon steak.
4. If necessary, use toothpicks to secure the bacon.
5. Turn the heat up to medium-high in a skillet.
6. After the skillet is hot, add the filet mignon steaks wrapped in bacon and sear them for about two minutes on each side or until the bacon begins to brown.
7. Move the sear-crusted filet mignon steaks to a baking tray.
8. After preheating the oven, put the baking dish inside and bake the filet mignon steaks for 10 to 12 minutes or until they are cooked to your preferred doneness.
9. After the filet mignons are cooked (to your preference), put them out of the oven and allow them to rest for a short while.
10. Before serving, take out the toothpicks.

FILET MIGNON
WITH TRUFFLE BUTTER

SERVING 2
PREP TIME: 10 MIN
COOK TIME: 10 MIN

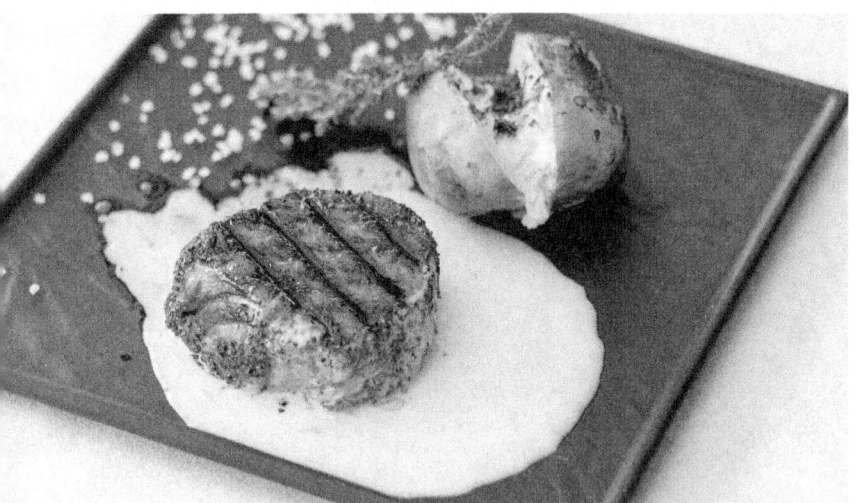

Juicy filet mignon steaks topped with decadent truffle butter, elevating the flavor to new heights. This dish is a true indulgence for steak lovers.

INGREDIENTS

- 2 filet mignon steaks, about 6 ounces each
- 2 tablespoons truffle butter
- Salt and black pepper to taste

NUTRITIONAL INFO

Cal 400 • Fat 30 g • Carb 0 g • Protein 30 g

INSTRUCTIONS

1. Remove the filet mignon steaks from the refrigerator and allow them to chill to room temperature for approximately half an hour. This promotes uniform cooking.
2. Turn up the heat on your grill or grill pan.
3. Season each filet mignon steak with salt and black pepper on both sides.
4. Place the filet mignon steaks on the hot grill or grill pan, then cook until medium-rare or to your preferred level of doneness, which typically takes about 3-4 minutes on each side. It's important to adjust the cooking duration based on the thickness of the steaks and your desired doneness.
5. After the filet mignon steaks are cooked (to your preference), take them off the grill or grill pan and place them onto a platter.
6. Give the steaks a few minutes to rest.
7. While the steaks are still warm, top each filet mignon with a tablespoon of truffle butter, allowing the butter to melt gently over the steaks.

RIBEYE STEAK
WITH BLUE CHEESE BUTTER

SERVING 2
PREP TIME: 10 MIN
COOK TIME: 10 MIN

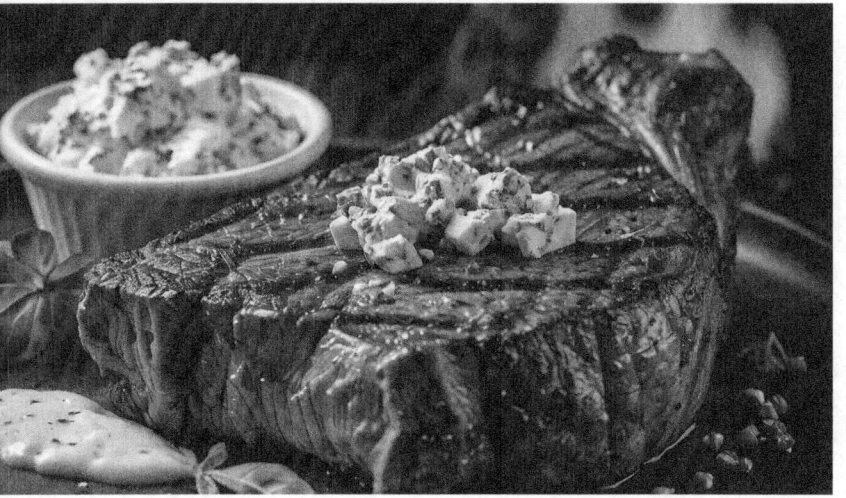

A juicy ribeye steak, cooked perfectly and served with a flavorful blue cheese butter topping. This combination offers a burst of flavors that steak enthusiasts will love.

INGREDIENTS

- 2 ribeye steaks, about 8 ounces each
- 2 tablespoons blue cheese, crumbled
- 2 tablespoons butter, softened
- Salt and black pepper to taste

NUTRITIONAL INFO

Cal 600 • Fat 45 g • Carb 2 g • Protein 45 g

ALLERGEN INFO

INSTRUCTIONS

1. Remove the ribeye steaks from the refrigerator and allow them to come to room temperature for approximately half an hour. This promotes uniform cooking.
2. Using a small bowl, thoroughly combine the crumbled blue cheese and softened butter.
3. Use salt and black pepper to season each ribeye steak on both sides.
4. Turn up the heat on your grill or grill pan.
5. Arrange the ribeye steaks on the hot grill or grill pan and cook for medium-rare or until desired doneness, about 4–5 minutes on each side. We recommend adjusting the cooking time according to the thickness and doneness you like the most.
6. After the ribeye steaks are cooked to your preference, remove them from the grill or grill pan and place them on a plate.
7. Give the steaks a few minutes to rest.
8. While the steaks are still warm, top each one with a generous dollop of blue cheese butter, allowing the butter to melt gently over the meat.

BEEF TENDERLOIN MEDALLIONS WITH PEPPERCORN SAUCE

SERVING 2
PREP TIME: 10 MIN
COOK TIME: 15 MIN

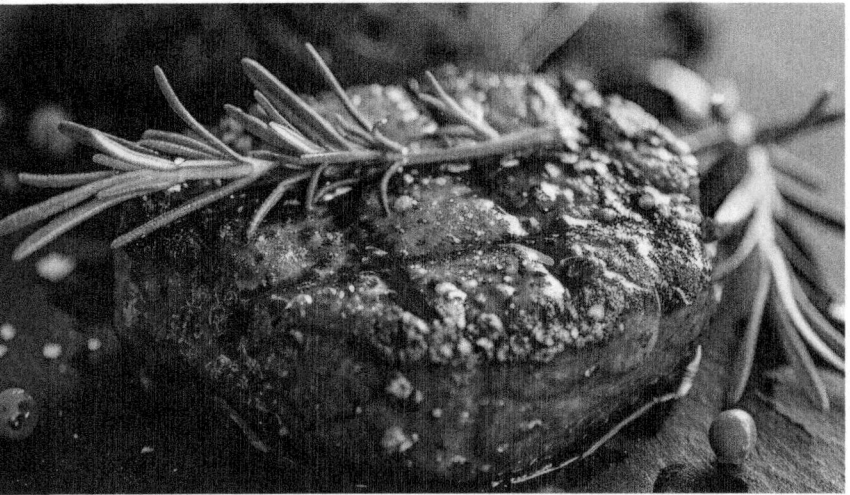

Tender beef medallions served with a creamy and peppery sauce. This elegant dish is perfect for a sophisticated dinner.

INGREDIENTS

- 2 beef tenderloin medallions, about 6 ounces each
- 1/2 cup heavy cream
- 2 tablespoons whole peppercorns
- Salt to taste
- 2 tablespoons butter or ghee

NUTRITIONAL INFO

Cal 500 • Fat 40 g • Carb 0 g • Protein 30 g

ALLERGEN INFO

INSTRUCTIONS

1. Crush all the peppercorns with a mortar and pestle, or place them in a zip-lock bag and crush them (use a rolling pin).
2. Season the beef tenderloin medallions with salt on both sides.
3. Heat the butter or ghee in a skillet over medium-high heat.
4. When the skillet is heated enough, add the beef tenderloin medallions and cook for 3-4 minutes on each side for medium-rare or until desired doneness. We recommend adjusting the cooking time according to the thickness of the medallions and your desired level of doneness.
5. Remove the cooked beef tenderloin medallions from the skillet and transfer them to a plate. Cover loosely with foil to keep warm.
6. In the same skillet, reduce the heat to medium and add the crushed pepper-corns. Cook and stir for 1-2 minutes until it gives off a pleasant aroma.
7. Pour in the heavy cream and stir to combine with the peppercorns. Let the sauce simmer for a while (3-4 minutes) until it thickens slightly.
8. Once the sauce has thickened, return the beef tenderloin medallions to the skillet and coat them with the peppercorn sauce.
9. Cook for an additional minute, ensuring the beef tenderloin medallions are heated through and coated evenly with the sauce.
10. Take the skillet off the heat and transfer the beef tenderloin medallions with peppercorn sauce to serving plates.

BEEF HEART STEAKS

SERVING 2
PREP TIME: 10 MIN
COOK TIME: 15 MIN

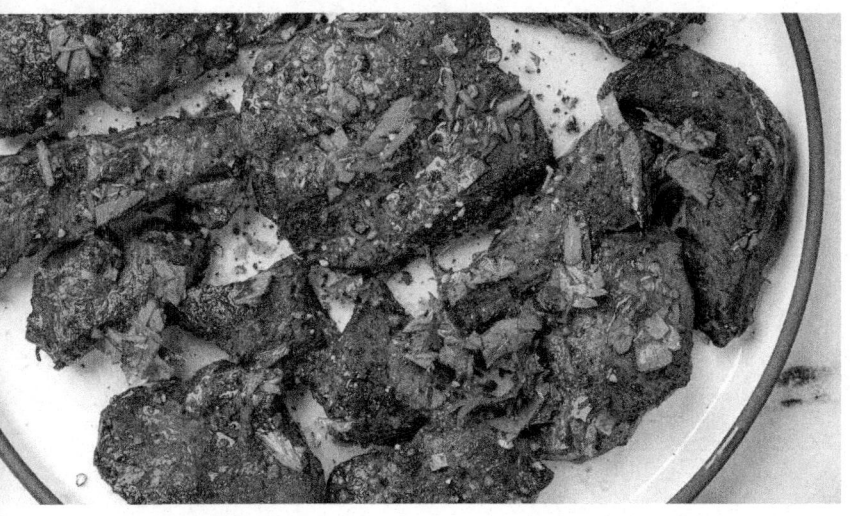

Rich and flavorful beef heart steaks grilled to perfection. A nutrient-dense option for those looking to explore organ meats.

INGREDIENTS

- 1 beef heart
- Salt and black pepper to taste
- Beef tallow for cooking

NUTRITIONAL INFO

Cal 250 • Fat 15 g • Carb 0 g • Protein 30 g

INSTRUCTIONS

1. Dry the beef with paper towels heart after rinsing it under cold water.
2. Remove any extra fat or connective tissue from the beef heart using a sharp knife.
3. Cut the beef heart into thick slices (1/2 to 3/4 inch).
4. Lightly season both sides of the beef heart slices with salt and black pepper.
5. Place a grill pan or skillet over medium-high heat and drizzle with either beef stock or olive oil.
6. After heating the skillet, put the beef heart slices in a single layer, taking care not to cover the entire surface of the pan.
7. Bake the beef heart steaks on each side for five to seven minutes or until they are cooked through and browned on the outside to your preferred doneness. For medium-rare, the interior temperature needs to be at least 145°F (63°C).
8. Take out the steaks from the skillet and allow them to settle for a short while before serving.

BAKED BEEF CHOPS
WITH MAYONNAISE AND CHEESE

SERVING 2
PREP TIME: 15 MIN
COOK TIME: 25 MIN

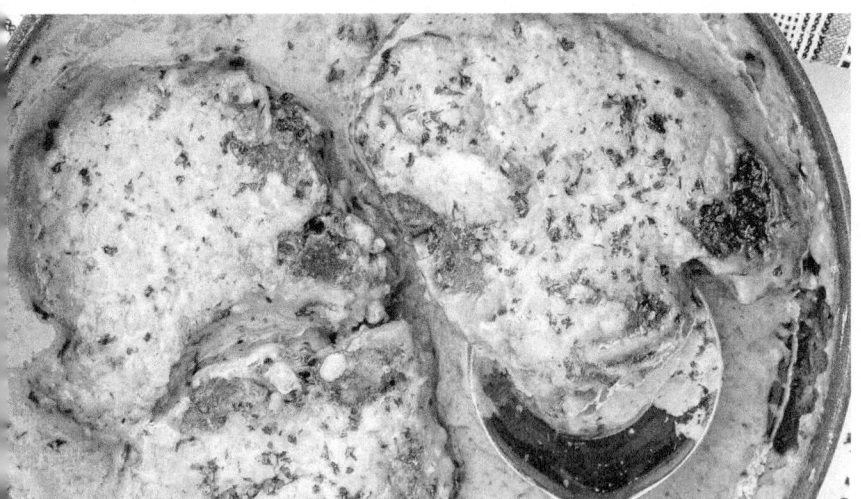

Juicy beef chops baked with a creamy layer of mayonnaise and melted cheese. This dish is both indulgent and satisfying, perfect for a hearty meal.

INGREDIENTS

- 2 beef chops (approximately 8 oz each)
- 4 tablespoons carnivore mayonnaise
- 1/2 cup shredded cheese (cheddar, mozzarella, or your choice)
- Salt, to taste
- Freshly ground black pepper (as much as preferred)

INSTRUCTIONS

1. Commence by preheating your oven to 375°F (190°C).
2. Season the beef chops with salt and freshly ground black pepper on both sides.
3. Spread 2 tablespoons of carnivore mayonnaise evenly over each beef chop.
4. Sprinkle 1/4 cup of shredded cheese over each beef chop, ensuring an even coating.
5. Place the beef chops on a baking sheet or dish.
6. Please bake the dish in the preheated oven until the beef reaches your preferred level of doneness and the cheese is melted and has a golden brown color.
7. Allow the beef chops to rest briefly before serving.

NUTRITIONAL INFO

Cal 650 • Fat 50 g • Carb 1 g • Protein 50 g

ALLERGEN INFO

PORK

- 74 PORK CHOP WITH SMOKED BACON BUTTER
- 75 PORK TENDERLOIN MEDALLIONS WITH SAGE BROWN BUTTER
- 76 CARNIVORE PORK STEW
- 77 CARNIVORE PORK STROGANOFF STYLE
- 78 BAKED PORK RIBS
- 79 PORK CUTLETS
- 80 CARNIVORE PORK SKEWERS
- 81 PORK CURLS WITH GRUYÈRE CHEESE
- 82 ROASTED PORK KNUCKLE
- 83 BAKED PORK BELLY
- 84 PORK AND SMOKED BACON CASSEROLE WITH EGGS
- 85 STEWED PORK IN SOUR CREAM SAUCE

PORK CHOP WITH
SMOKED BACON BUTTER

SERVING 2
PREP TIME: 10 MIN
COOK TIME: 25 MIN

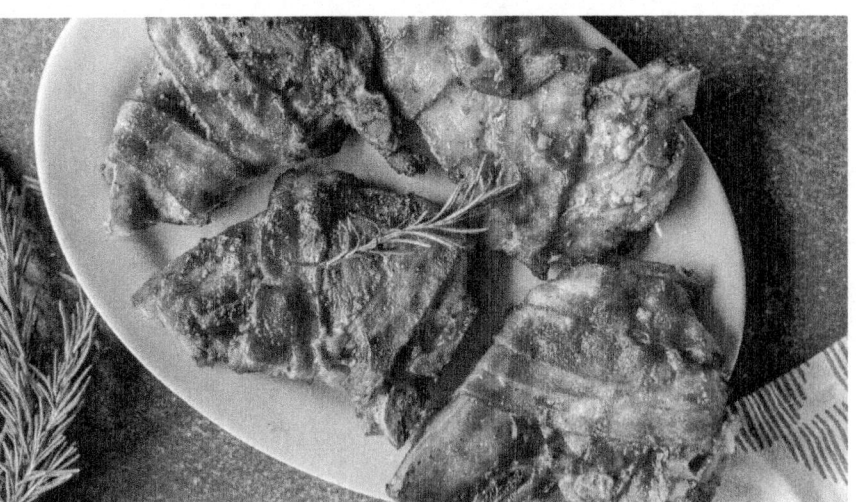

Juicy pork chops grilled to perfection and topped with rich smoked bacon butter. This dish offers a savory and satisfying meal with a smoky twist.

INGREDIENTS

- 2 pork chops
- 4 slices of smoked bacon
- 4 tablespoons butter
- Salt and black pepper to taste

NUTRITIONAL INFO

Cal 400 • Fat 30 g • Carb 0 g • Protein 30 g

ALLERGEN INFO

INSTRUCTIONS

1. Heat your skillet or grill to a medium-high temperature.
2. Season the pork chops with a classical mix of pepper and salt on both sides.
3. Grill or skillet-cook pork chops for 5 to 7 minutes on each side or until cooked through and the internal temperature is 145°F (63°C).
4. In a separate skillet, cook the bacon slices until crispy while the pork chops. Take the bacon off the skillet and let it cool a little.
5. Cut the bacon into little pieces as soon as it's cool enough to handle.
6. Melt the butter over low heat (use a small saucepan).
7. Stir to combine the chopped bacon with the melted butter.
8. Allow the flavors to mingle together by cooking the bacon-butter combination for two to three minutes.
9. After the pork chops are cooked, take them off the grill or skillet and place them on a dish for serving.
10. Drizzle the smoked bacon butter over the roasts.

PORK TENDERLOIN MEDALLIONS
WITH SAGE BROWN BUTTER

SERVING 2
PREP TIME: 10 MIN
COOK TIME: 15 MIN

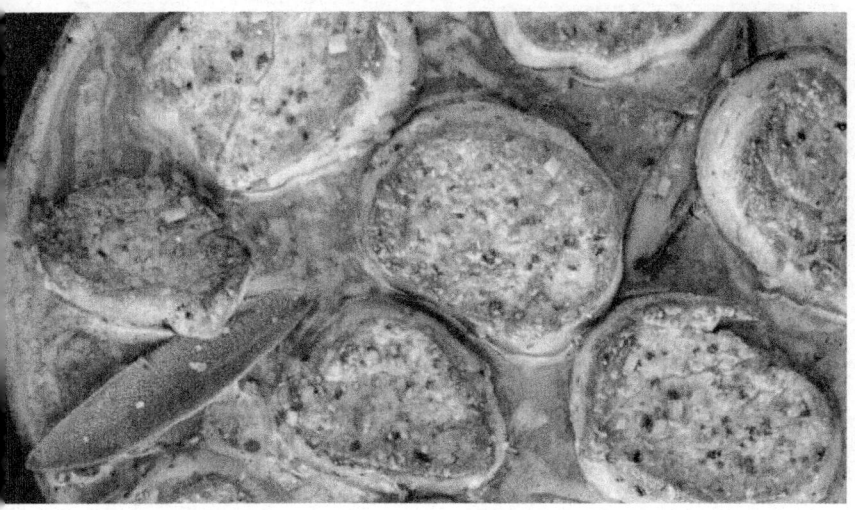

Tender pork medallions cooked in a fragrant sage brown butter sauce. This elegant dish is perfect for a sophisticated yet easy-to-prepare dinner.

INGREDIENTS

- 1 pork tenderloin, about 1 lb
- 8-10 fresh sage leaves
- 4 tablespoons butter
- Salt and black pepper to taste

NUTRITIONAL INFO

Cal 400 • Fat 25 g • Carb 0 g • Protein 35 g

ALLERGEN INFO

INSTRUCTIONS

1. Cut the pork tenderloin into medallions, each measuring about one inch thick. Season the medallions on both sides with black pepper and salt.
2. Set the heat up to medium-high and add butter (two tablespoons) to a pan.
3. Add the pork tenderloin medallions to the skillet when the butter melts and becomes flavorful. Bake for approximately 3–4 minutes on each side or until well-cooked and golden. The interior temperature ought to be 145°F, or 63°C.
4. Make the sage-brown butter while the roast is cooking. You can melt the remaining two butter over medium heat (in a separate small pot).
5. Add the fresh sage leaves to the saucepan when the butter has melted. Cook for one to two minutes or until the butter takes on a golden brown hue and the sage leaves become crispy.
6. Set aside the sage leaves from the browned butter.
7. Take the cooked pork tenderloin medallions from the skillet and place them on a tray for serving.
8. Drizzle the steak tenderloin medallions with the sage-infused butter.

CARNIVORE PORK STEW

> **SERVING 2**
> PREP TIME: 10 MIN
> COOK TIME: 2-3 HOURS

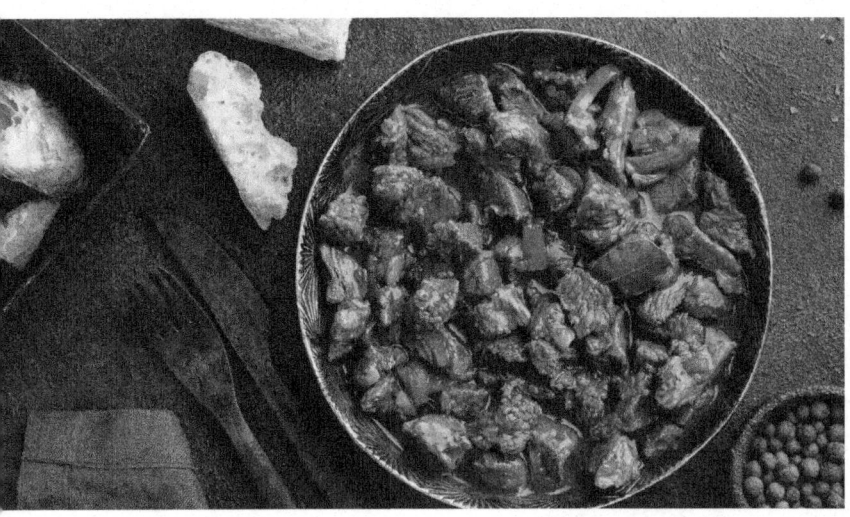

A hearty pork stew slow-cooked in beef bone broth, seasoned with salt and pepper. This comforting dish is rich in flavor and perfect for a nourishing meal.

INGREDIENTS

- 1/2 lb pork belly or shoulder, cut into bite-sized pieces
- 1 cup beef bone broth or water
- Salt and black pepper
- Optional: herbs or spices such as rosemary, thyme, garlic powder)

NUTRITIONAL INFO

Cal 250 • Fat 15 g • Carb 0 g • Protein 15 g

INSTRUCTIONS

1. Set your oven to preheat to 300°F (150°C).
2. Combine the pork pieces and beef bone broth (or water) in a small oven-safe pot or Dutch oven.
3. Season with black pepper or salt (to taste).
4. Optional: Add any desired herbs and spices for flavoring, such as rosemary, thyme, or garlic powder.
5. Cover the pot and put it in the preheated oven.
6. Let the stew cook in the oven for 2-3 hours or until the pork is tender and fully cooked.
7. Once the stew is done, take it off the oven and cool it slightly before serving.
8. Taste and add the seasoning if necessary.

CARNIVORE PORK
STROGANOFF STYLE

SERVING 2
PREP TIME: 10 MIN
COOK TIME: 25 MIN

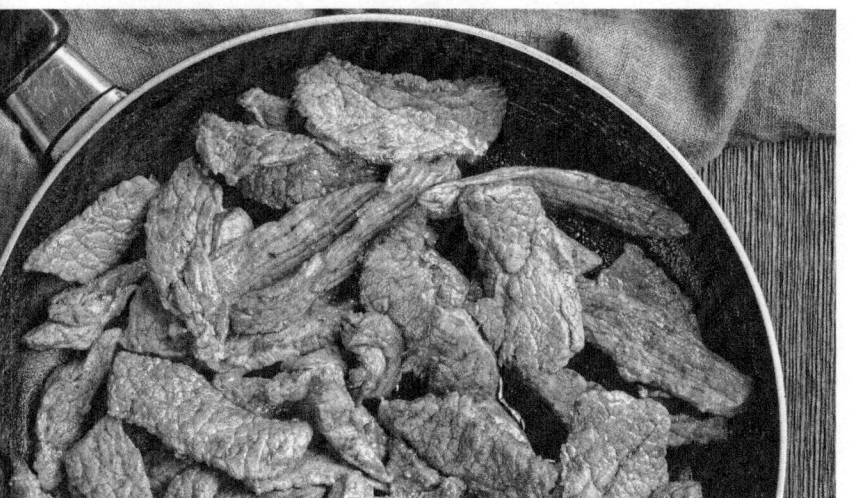

Thinly sliced pork loin cooked with crispy bacon and a creamy beef bone broth sauce. This dish is a carnivore-friendly take on the classic stroganoff.

INGREDIENTS

- 1/2 lb pork loin or pork tenderloin, thinly sliced
- 2 slices bacon, chopped
- 1/2 cup beef bone broth or water
- 1/4 cup heavy cream
- 1 tablespoon butter
- Salt and black pepper to taste

NUTRITIONAL INFO

Cal 200 • Fat 15 g • Carb 0 g • Protein 15 g

ALLERGEN INFO

INSTRUCTIONS

1. In a skillet, cook the chopped bacon over medium heat until crispy. Remove the bacon from the skillet and set it aside.
2. Add the thinly sliced pork loin or tenderloin in the same skillet. Cook the food until it is browned on all sides and cooked through, which should take approximately 5 to 7 minutes.
3. Remove the cooked pork from the skillet and set it aside with the bacon.
4. Pour the beef bone broth (or water) into the skillet and use a spatula to scrape up any browned bits from the bottom, making sure to deglaze the pan.
5. You can combine the heavy cream and butter and then heat the mixture until it simmers.
6. After the pork and bacon are cooked, put them back in the skillet and let them simmer for 5 to 10 minutes until the sauce thickens slightly.
7. Season with pepper and salt (to taste).

BAKED PORK RIBS

> **SERVING 2**
> PREP TIME: 10 MIN
> COOK TIME: 2 HOURS

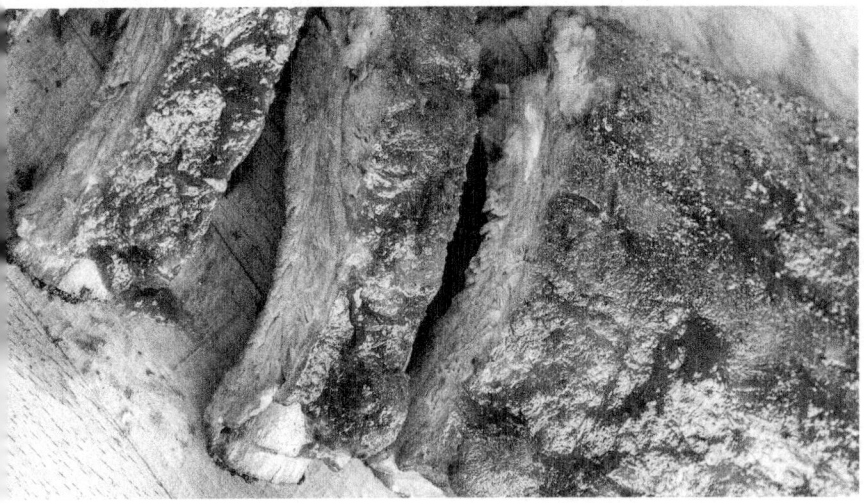

Tender and flavorful pork ribs are baked until the meat falls off the bone. These ribs are a perfect main course for a hearty meal.

INGREDIENTS

- 2 lbs pork ribs
- 1 tablespoon salt
- 1 teaspoon black pepper

NUTRITIONAL INFO

Cal 700 • Fat 55 g • Carb 0 g • Protein 50 g

INSTRUCTIONS

1. Commence by preheating your oven to 300°F (150°C).
2. Take the membrane off the back of the ribs for better tenderness.
3. Season the ribs with pepper and salt.
4. Place the ribs on a tray (lined with aluminum foil) or in a roasting pan.
5. Cover the ribs with aluminum foil to keep them moist.
6. Bake in the oven (preheated) for 2 hours or until the meat is so tender that it easily pulls away from the bone.
7. For a crispier finish, you can choose to remove the foil and raise the oven temperature to 425°F (220°C).
8. Broil the ribs for 5-10 minutes, keeping a close eye on them to prevent burning.
9. Let the ribs rest briefly before slicing and serving.

PORK CUTLETS

SERVING 2
PREP TIME: 10 MIN
COOK TIME: 2 HOURS

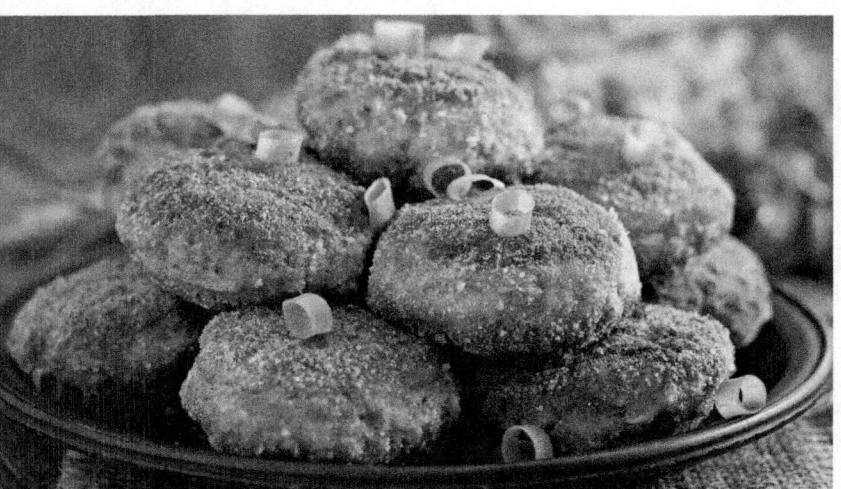

Golden brown pork cutlets fried in pork lard or beef tallow. These cutlets are crispy on the outside and juicy on the inside, making for a delightful meal.

INGREDIENTS

- 1 lb minced pork
- 1 large egg
- Salt, to taste
- Freshly ground black pepper (as much as preferred)
- 2 tablespoons pork lard or beef tallow

NUTRITIONAL INFO

Cal 450 • Fat 30 g • Carb 0 g • Protein 40 g

ALLERGEN INFO

INSTRUCTIONS

1. Combine the minced pork, egg, pepper, and salt in a mixing bowl. Mix until well combined.
2. Shape the mixture into small cutlets, approximately 2-3 inches in diameter.
3. Heat the pork lard or beef tallow in a large pan (over medium-high heat) until it is fully melted and hot.
4. Add the cutlets to the frying pan. Fry on each side for about 4-5 minutes or until the cutlets are golden brown and cooked through. Ensure the internal temperature of the cutlets reaches 160°F (71°C).
5. Remove the cutlets from the frying pan and let them rest for a few minutes before serving.

CARNIVORE PORK SKEWERS

> **SERVING 2**
> PREP TIME: 10 MIN
> COOK TIME: 15 MIN

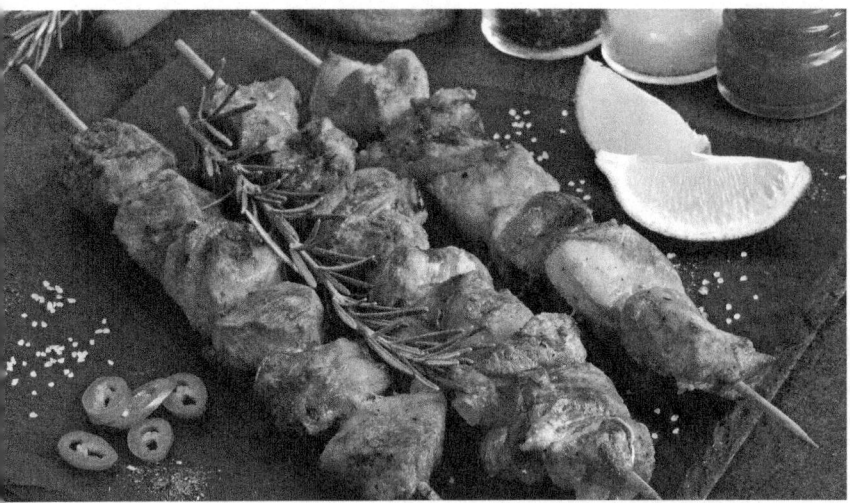

Seasoned pork cubes grilled to perfection on skewers. These skewers are a tasty and convenient way to enjoy pork.

INGREDIENTS

- 1 lb pork loin or tenderloin, cut into cube shape
- Salt, to taste
- Freshly ground black pepper (as much as preferred)
- 2 tablespoons pork lard or beef tallow, melted

NUTRITIONAL INFO

Cal 500 • Fat 35 g • Carb 0 g • Protein 45 g

INSTRUCTIONS

1. Make sure to preheat your grill or grill pan to medium-high heat.
2. Season the pork cubes with salt and freshly ground black pepper.
3. Thread the seasoned pork cubes onto skewers, evenly distributing them.
4. Brush the grill grates with a bit of melted pork lard or beef tallow to prevent sticking.
5. Place the pork skewers on the preheated grill or grill pan.
6. Grill for 6-8 minutes on each side or until the pork is cooked through and has grill marks.
7. Remove the pork skewers from the grill and let them rest for a few minutes.

PORK CURLS
WITH GRUYÈRE CHEESE

SERVING 2
PREP TIME: 10 MIN
COOK TIME: 20 MIN

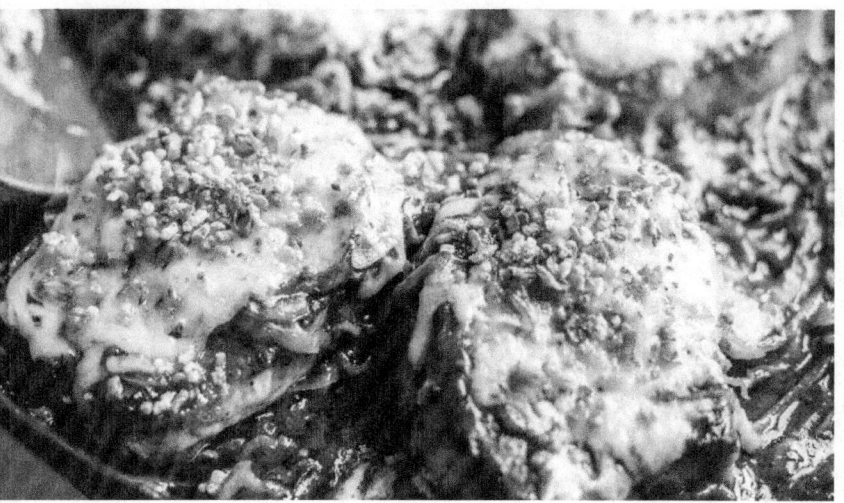

Thinly sliced pork loin rolled up and baked with shredded Gruyère cheese. This dish combines savory pork with creamy melted cheese for a delectable treat.

INGREDIENTS

- 1 lb pork loin, thinly sliced into strips
- Salt, to taste
- Freshly ground black pepper (as much as preferred)
- 1 cup shredded Gruyère cheese

NUTRITIONAL INFO

Cal 600 • Fat 45 g • Carb 0 g • Protein 50 g

ALLERGEN INFO

INSTRUCTIONS

1. Commence by preheating your oven to 375°F (190°C).
2. Season the thinly sliced pork loin strips with salt and freshly ground black pepper.
3. Roll each pork strip up tightly to form a curl. If necessary, secure the end with a toothpick.
4. Position the rolled pork curls on a baking tray (lined either with aluminum foil or parchment paper), ensuring they are the same side down and not touching each other.
5. Sprinkle the shredded Gruyère cheese evenly over the pork curls, ensuring each one is generously coated.
6. Cook the dish in the oven that has been preheated for 15-20 minutes, or until the pork is fully cooked and the cheese has melted and become bubbly with a golden brown crust.
7. Remove the pork curls from the oven and let them cool for a few minutes before serving.

ROASTED PORK KNUCKLE

SERVING 2
PREP TIME: 10 MIN
COOK TIME: 2 HOURS

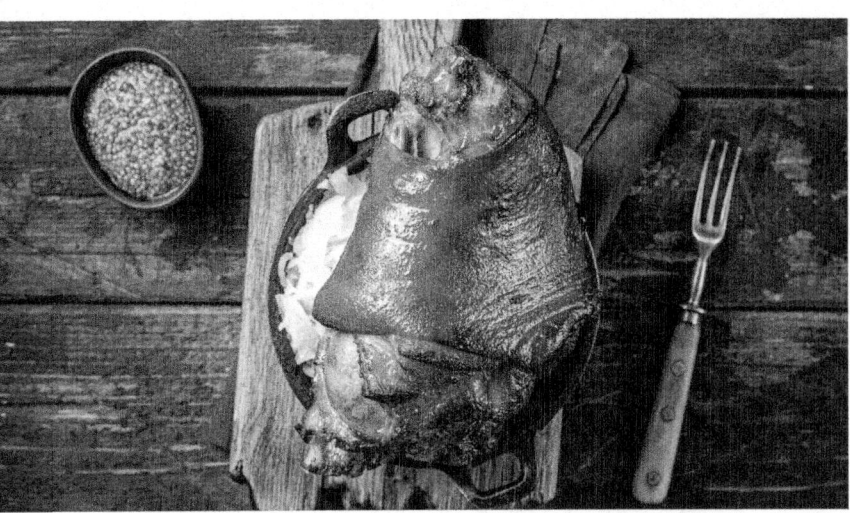

Crispy-skinned pork knuckle roasted to perfection, offering tender meat inside. This dish is both impressive and delicious, perfect for a hearty meal.

INGREDIENTS

- 2 pork knuckles (approximately 1 lb each)
- Salt, to taste
- Freshly ground black pepper (as much as preferred)

NUTRITIONAL INFO

Cal 800 • Fat 60 g • Carb 0 g • Protein 60 g

INSTRUCTIONS

1. Commence by preheating your oven to 350°F (175°C).
2. Make little cuts on the pork knuckles' skin in a crisscross pattern (with a knife). This helps the fat to be rendered and the skin to become crispy during roasting.
3. Season the pork knuckles generously with salt and freshly ground black pepper, rubbing the seasoning into the skin and meat.
4. Place the seasoned pork knuckles on a roasting tray or in a baking dish, ensuring they are not touching each other.
5. Put the dish into the oven (preheated) and roast for roughly 2 hours, or until the skin achieves a crispy texture and the meat becomes tender and thoroughly cooked. Raise the temperature inside to (at least) 160°F (71°C).
6. Remove the roasted pork knuckles from the oven and let them rest for a few minutes before serving.

BAKED PORK BELLY

SERVING 2
PREP TIME: 10 MIN
COOK TIME: 30 MIN

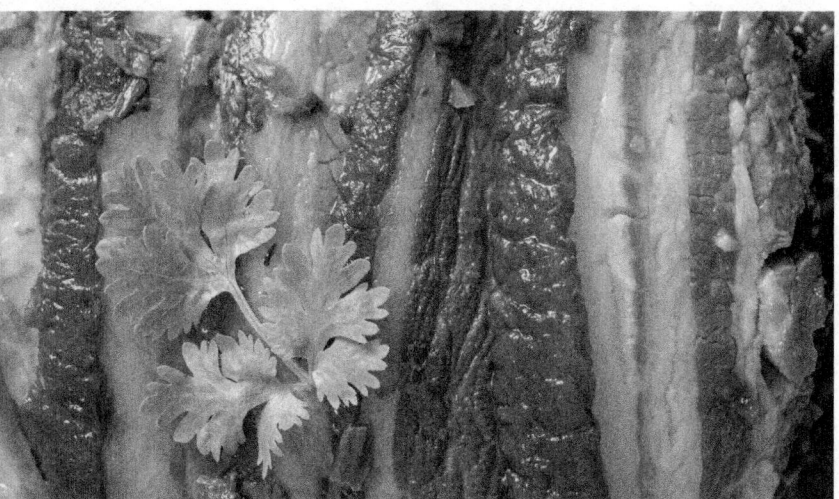

Pork belly is cooked until the skin is crispy and the meat is tender, resulting in a rich and flavorful dish. This indulgent dish is a carnivore favorite, offering a melt-in-your-mouth experience.

INGREDIENTS

- 1 lb pork belly
- Salt, to taste
- Freshly ground black pepper (as much as preferred)
- 1 cup water

NUTRITIONAL INFO

Cal 800 • Fat 70 g • Carb 0 g • Protein 40 g

INSTRUCTIONS

1. Commence by preheating your oven to 325°F (160°C).
2. Begin by washing the pork belly under cold water and then drying it thoroughly with paper towels. Make cuts on the pork belly skin with a sharp knife (cuts should be about 1/4 inch apart). This helps the fat render during baking.
3. Season the pork belly generously with salt and freshly ground black pepper, rubbing the seasoning into the skin and meat.
4. Add enough water to cover the seasoned pork belly in a large pot. Start by heating the water until it boils over high heat and put the heat down (to medium-low) and for next 30 minutes let it simmer. This helps to render out some of the fat and tenderize the meat.
5. Transfer the parboiled pork belly to a roasting tray or baking dish, skin side up.
6. Pour some water (a cup) into the tray to prevent the pork belly from drying out during baking.
7. Bake in the oven that has been preheated for around 2 hours or until the meat becomes tender, the skin is crispy, and the belly is fully cooked.
8. Remove the baked pork belly from the oven and let it rest for a few minutes before slicing and serving.
9. You can serve the baked pork belly with your favorite carnivore-friendly sauce or enjoy it as is.

PORK AND SMOKED
BACON CASSEROLE WITH EGGS

SERVING 2
PREP TIME: 20 MIN
COOK TIME: 1 HOUR

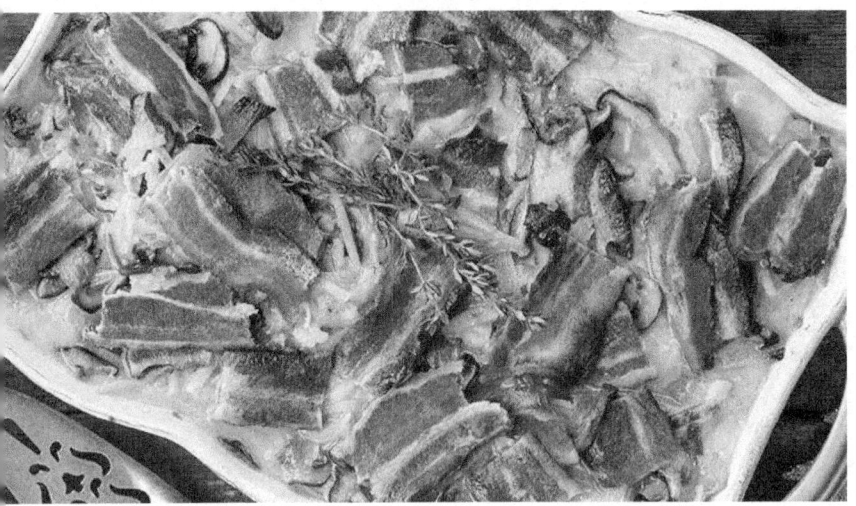

A savory casserole featuring diced pork shoulder, smoked bacon, and beaten eggs. This dish is baked to perfection, providing a protein-packed meal.

INGREDIENTS

- 1 lb pork shoulder, diced
- 6 slices smoked bacon, chopped
- Salt, to taste
- Freshly ground black pepper (as much as preferred)
- 4 large eggs, beaten
- 1 cup beef or bone broth
- 1 tablespoon beef tallow or pork lard
- Optional: chopped fresh herbs for garnish

NUTRITIONAL INFO

Cal 720 • Fat 57 g • Carb 0 g • Protein 53 g

ALLERGEN INFO

INSTRUCTIONS

1. Commence by preheating your oven to 350°F (175°C).
2. Season the diced pork shoulder and chopped smoked bacon with salt and freshly ground black pepper.
3. Heat beef tallow or pork lard in a large ovenproof skillet or casserole dish over medium-high heat.
4. Add the diced pork shoulder and chopped smoked bacon to the skillet. Sear until browned (for about 5 minutes).
5. Pour the beef or bone broth into the skillet, stirring to combine, and deglaze the bottom of the pan.
6. Evenly pour the beaten eggs over the meat and bacon mixture in the skillet.
7. Cover the casserole dish or skillet with aluminum foil or a lid.
8. Transfer to the oven (preheated) and bake for 45 minutes to 1 hour, or until the pork is tender and cooked through and the eggs are set.
9. When cooked, take it off the oven and let it rest for a few minutes.

STEWED PORK IN SOUR
CREAM SAUCE

SERVING 2
PREP TIME: 20 MIN
COOK TIME: 1 HR 30 MIN

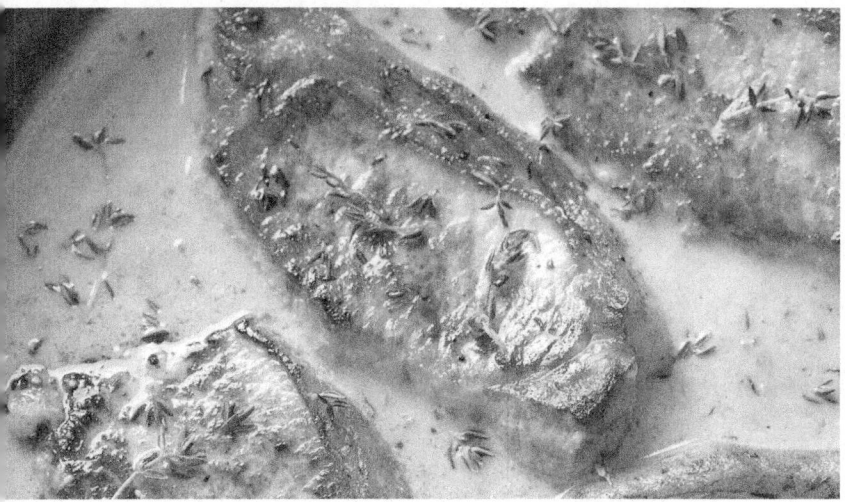

Tender pork shoulder stewed in a rich sour cream sauce. This dish is comforting and flavorful, perfect for a satisfying meal.

INGREDIENTS

- 1 lb pork shoulder, cubed
- Salt, to taste
- Freshly ground black pepper (as much as preferred)
- 2 tablespoons beef tallow or pork lard
- 1/2 cup beef or bone broth
- 1/2 cup sour cream

NUTRITIONAL INFO

Cal 600 • Fat 45 g • Carb 4 g • Protein 40 g

ALLERGEN INFO

INSTRUCTIONS

1. Season the cubed pork shoulder with salt and freshly ground black pepper to taste.
2. Heat beef tallow or pork lard in a skillet over medium-high heat.
3. Add the cubed pork shoulder to the skillet and brown it on all sides for about 5 minutes.
4. When adding the beef or bone broth to the skillet, remember to scrape off any browned bits found at the bottom of the pan.
5. Set the heat to low, cover the skillet, and simmer until the pork is tender and cooked through (for about 1 hour).
6. Stir in the sour cream until well combined.
7. Simmer for an additional 10-15 minutes, uncovered, allowing the sauce to thicken slightly.

POULTRY

87	BAKED CHICKEN WINGS
88	CHICKEN CONFIT
89	CHICKEN FINGERS
90	CHICKEN CORDON BLEU ROULADE
91	PROSCIUTTO-WRAPPED STUFFED TURKEY
92	TURKEY AND CHEESE GRILLED KEBABS
93	TURKEY MEATBALLS WITH CREAM SAUCE
94	CHICKEN MEATBALLS WITH CREAMY CHEESE SAUCE
95	ROAST GOOSE WITH SAGE AND THYME
96	DUCK ROULADE WITH FRENCH HERBS
97	CHICKEN CHEESE KEBAB
98	CHICKEN FRICASSEE WITH CREAMY DOR BLUE SAUCE

BAKED CHICKEN WINGS

> **SERVING 2**
> PREP TIME: 20 MIN
> COOK TIME: 45 MIN

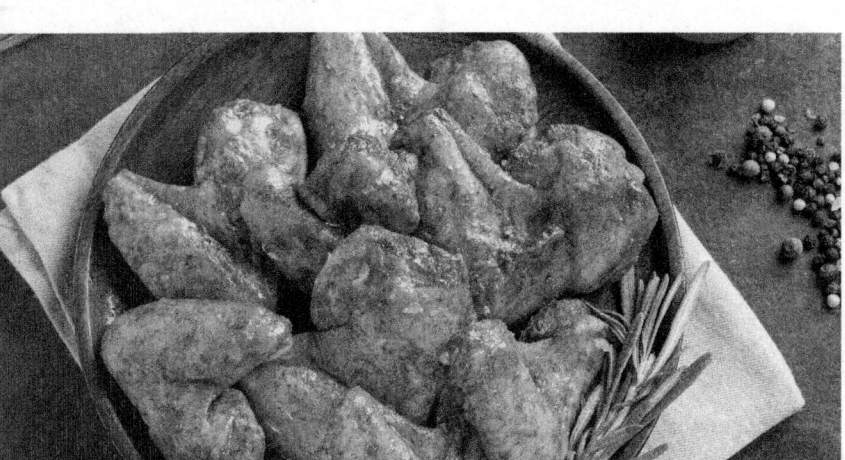

Crispy baked chicken wings seasoned with salt and pepper offer a simple yet flavorful snack or appetizer. They're perfect for game days or casual gatherings.

INGREDIENTS

- 1 lb chicken wings
- Salt, to taste
- Freshly ground black pepper (as much as preferred)
- 1 tablespoon beef tallow or pork lard (for greasing)

NUTRITIONAL INFO

Cal 400 • Fat 30 g • Carb 0 g • Protein 35 g

INSTRUCTIONS

1. Commence by preheating your oven to 425°F (220°C).
2. Wash the chicken wings with cold water and dry them with paper towels.
3. Add seasoning to the chicken wings (salt and freshly ground black pepper to taste).
4. Grease a baking sheet with beef tallow or pork lard to prevent sticking.
5. Arrange (in a single layer) the seasoned chicken wings on the baking tray and make sure to leave space between each wing.
6. Pop the baking sheet into the oven that has already been preheated and let the wings bake for 45 minutes. Make sure to flip the wings halfway through the cooking time so that they are evenly golden brown and crispy.
7. After the chicken wings have finished cooking, take them out of the oven and let them cool for a few minutes before serving.

CHICKEN CONFIT

SERVING 2
PREP TIME: 10 MIN
COOK TIME: 3 HRS 15 MIN

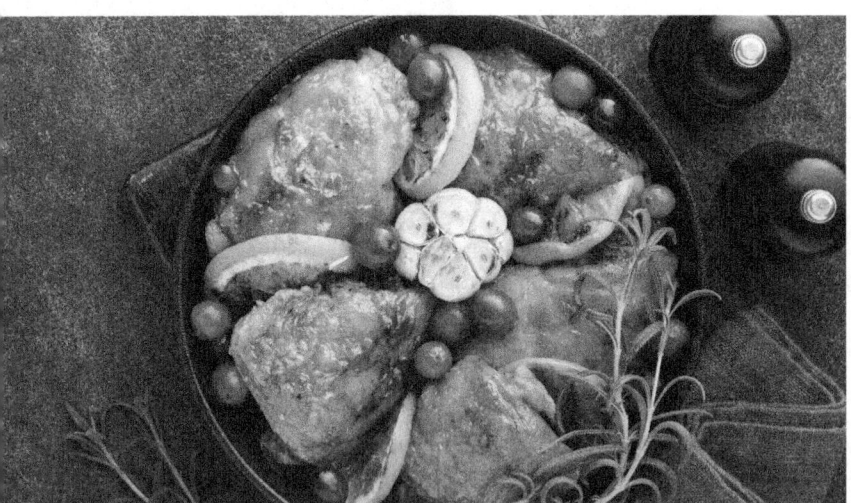

Tender chicken leg quarters are slowly cooked in duck fat with garlic and thyme. This rich, flavorful dish makes for a gourmet meal.

INGREDIENTS

- 2 chicken leg quarters, skin-on
- 2 cups duck fat or rendered chicken fat
- 2 cloves garlic, smashed
- 2 sprigs of fresh thyme
- 1 bay leaf
- Salt and black pepper to taste

NUTRITIONAL INFO

Cal 500 • Fat 40 g • Carb 0 g • Protein 25 g

INSTRUCTIONS

1. Commence by preheating your oven to 250°F (120°C).
2. Season the chicken leg quarters generously with salt and black pepper.
3. Arrange the chicken leg quarters in a single layer in a small ovenproof pot or Dutch oven.
4. Add the smashed garlic cloves, fresh thyme sprigs, and bay leaf to the pot, distributing them evenly around the chicken.
5. Pour the duck fat or rendered chicken fat over the chicken leg quarters, ensuring they are completely submerged.
6. Cover the pot and place it in the oven (preheated). Cook until the chicken is very tender so that it almost falls off the bone (for 2.5 or 3 hours).
7. When cooked, take the pot off the oven and let the chicken cool slightly in the fat.
8. Gently separate the chicken leg quarters from the excess fat and put them on a baking tray (covered with foil or parchment paper).
9. Optionally, increase the oven temperature to 425°F (220°C) and roast the chicken leg quarters for about 10-15 minutes to crisp up the skin.

CHICKEN FINGERS

> **SERVING 2**
> PREP TIME: 15 MIN
> COOK TIME: 15 MIN

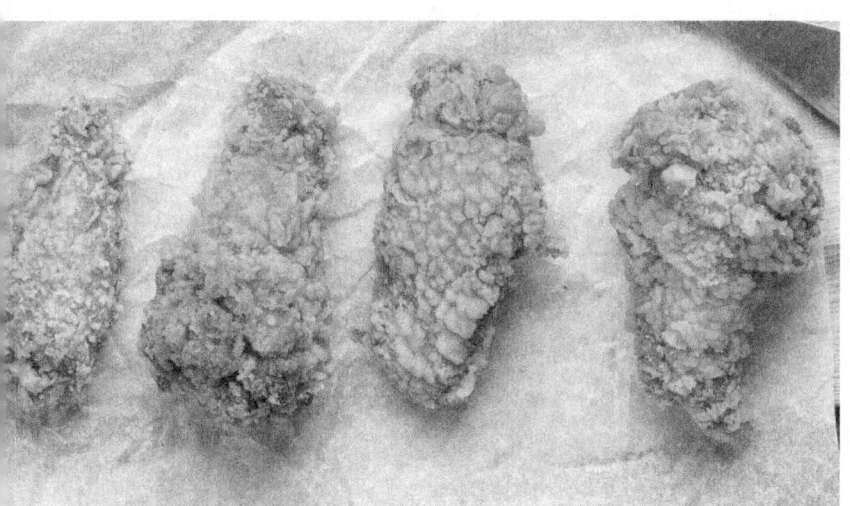

Juicy chicken breast strips coated in Parmesan cheese and fried until golden brown. A delicious and kid-friendly option for a quick meal or snack.

INGREDIENTS

- 2 boneless, skinless chicken breasts
- Salt and black pepper to taste
- 1 cup grated Parmesan cheese
- 2 eggs
- 1/2 teaspoon garlic powder
- 1/2 teaspoon paprika
- Cooking oil for frying

NUTRITIONAL INFO

Cal 300 • Fat 20 g • Carb 0 g • Protein 25 g

ALLERGEN INFO

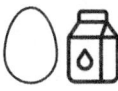

INSTRUCTIONS

1. Cut the chicken breasts into strips, about 1 inch wide.
2. Season the chicken strips with a dash of black pepper and a pinch of salt.
3. In a shallow dish, mix the grated Parmesan cheese, garlic powder, and paprika.
4. Beat the eggs in another dish.
5. Dip the chicken strips into the eggs, allowing any excess to drip off.
6. Dredge the chicken strip in the Parmesan cheese mixture, pressing gently to coat it evenly.
7. Heat cooking oil in a skillet over medium-high heat.
8. Once the oil is hot, carefully add the coated chicken strips to the skillet, ensuring not to overcrowd the pan.
9. Cook the chicken strips for about 3-4 minutes on each side or until they are golden brown and cooked through.
10. After cooking, take out the chicken strips from the skillet and put them on a plate (place paper towels on it to get rid of any extra oil).
11. Repeat the process with the remaining chicken strips.

CHICKEN CORDON BLEU ROULADE

SERVING 2
PREP TIME: 20 MIN
COOK TIME: 30 MIN

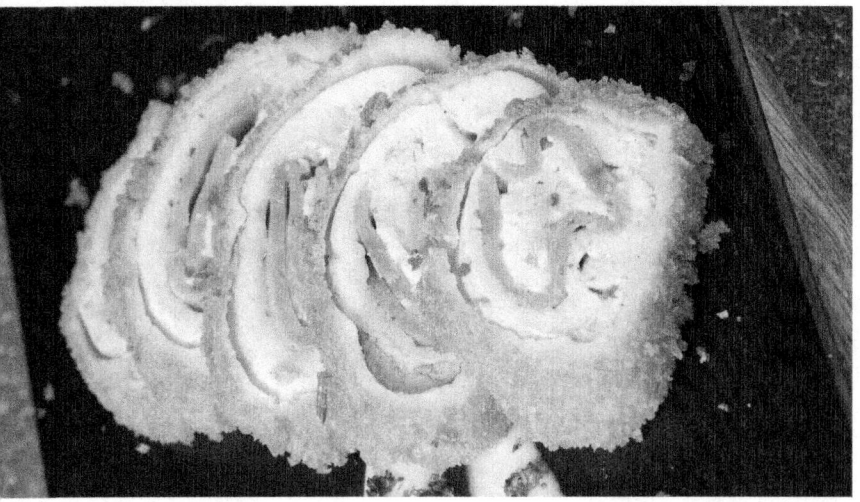

Rolled chicken breasts stuffed with ham and Swiss cheese, then baked to perfection. The timeless dish provides a delightful blend of flavors with each mouthful.

INGREDIENTS

- 2 boneless, skinless chicken breasts
- Salt and black pepper to taste
- 4 slices of ham
- 4 slices Swiss cheese
- 1/4 cup rendered bacon fat or lard
- Toothpicks

NUTRITIONAL INFO

Cal 400 • Fat 20 g • Carb 0 g • Protein 35 g

ALLERGEN INFO

INSTRUCTIONS

1. Commence by preheating your oven to 375°F (190°C).
2. Place one chicken breast between two sheets of plastic wrap. To make them evenly thick (about 1/4 inch), use a rolling pin or meat mallet to pound the chicken breast.
3. Season the pounded chicken breast with salt and black pepper.
4. Place two slices of ham and two slices of Swiss cheese on the chicken breast.
5. Starting from one end, roll up the chicken breast tightly, tucking in the filling as you go. Secure the roll with toothpicks.
6. Repeat the process with the remaining chicken breast and filling.
7. Heat rendered bacon fat or lard in an ovenproof skillet over medium-high heat.
8. Once the skillet is hot, add the chicken roulades and sear them until golden brown, about 2-3 minutes per side.
9. Put the skillet into the preheated oven and cook the chicken roulades for 20-25 minutes until they are cooked thoroughly and reach an internal temperature of 165°F (75°C).
10. Once cooked, remove the skillet from the oven and let the chicken roulades rest for a few minutes before slicing.
11. Remove the toothpicks from the chicken roulades and slice them into thick rounds.

PROSCIUTTO-WRAPPED
STUFFED TURKEY

SERVING 2
PREP TIME: 10 MIN
COOK TIME: 25 MIN

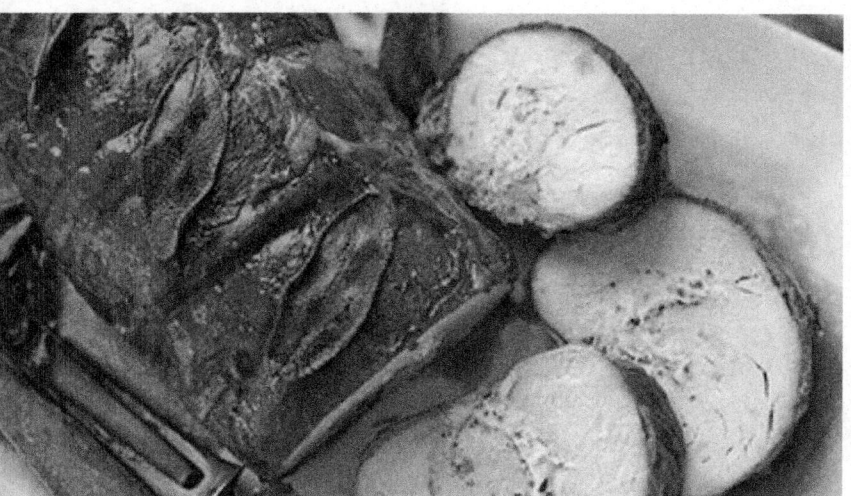

Turkey breast fillets stuffed with mozzarella cheese and wrapped in crispy prosciuttoThey are an elegant and satisfying dish for special occasions.

INGREDIENTS

- 2 turkey breast fillets
- Salt and black pepper to taste
- 4 slices prosciutto
- 1/2 cup shredded mozzarella cheese
- 2 tablespoons pork lard or beef tallow

NUTRITIONAL INFO

Cal 400 • Fat 20 g • Carb 0 g • Protein 45 g

ALLERGEN INFO

INSTRUCTIONS

1. Commence by preheating your oven to 375°F (190°C).
2. Lay each turkey breast fillet flat on a cutting board and season with salt and black pepper.
3. Divide the shredded mozzarella cheese evenly between the two turkey breast fillets, placing the filling on one side of each fillet.
4. Roll up each turkey breast fillet tightly, enclosing the filling. Wrap each rolled turkey breast fillet with 2 slices of prosciutto, ensuring they are fully covered.
5. Heat pork lard or beef tallow in an ovenproof skillet over medium-high heat.
6. When the skillet is hot, place the prosciutto-wrapped turkey breast fillets in it and sear them on all sides until the prosciutto is crispy and golden brown, about 2-3 minutes per side.
7. Place the skillet in the oven that has been preheated and cook the prosciutto-wrapped stuffed turkey breast fillets until cooked with an internal temperature of 165°F (75°C) (for 20-25 minutes).
8. Once cooked, remove the skillet from the oven and let the turkey breast fillets rest for a few minutes before slicing.

TURKEY AND CHEESE
GRILLED KEBABS

SERVING 2
PREP TIME: 15 MIN
COOK TIME: 10 MIN

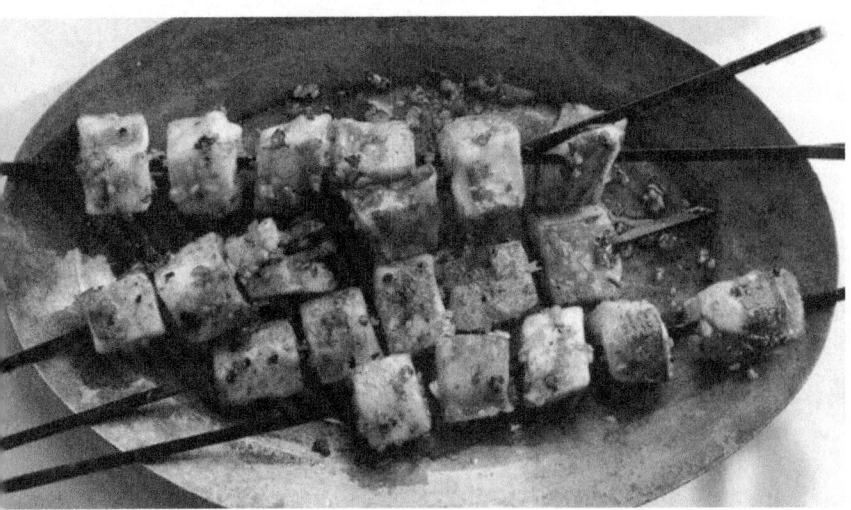

Tender turkey breast cubes and cheese grilled on skewers, creating a savory and fun meal. Perfect for barbecues or quick dinners.

INGREDIENTS

- 2 turkey breast fillets, cut into cubes
- Salt and black pepper to taste
- 4 slices cheddar or mozzarella cheese, cut into cubes
- Soaked wooden skewers

NUTRITIONAL INFO

Cal 400 • Fat 20 g • Carb 0 g • Protein 45 g

ALLERGEN INFO

INSTRUCTIONS

1. Preheat your grill to medium-high heat.
2. Season the turkey breast cubes with salt and black pepper.
3. Alternately thread the seasoned turkey cubes and cheese cubes onto the soaked wooden skewers, leaving a little space between each cube.
4. Brush the turkey and cheese kebabs with olive oil to prevent sticking.
5. Put the skewers on the grill and cook for 8-10 minutes, occasionally turning, until the turkey is cooked and has grill marks on all sides.
6. Once cooked, remove the kebabs from the grill and let them rest for a few minutes before serving.

TURKEY MEATBALLS
WITH CREAM SAUCE

SERVING 2
PREP TIME: 15 MIN
COOK TIME: 25 MIN

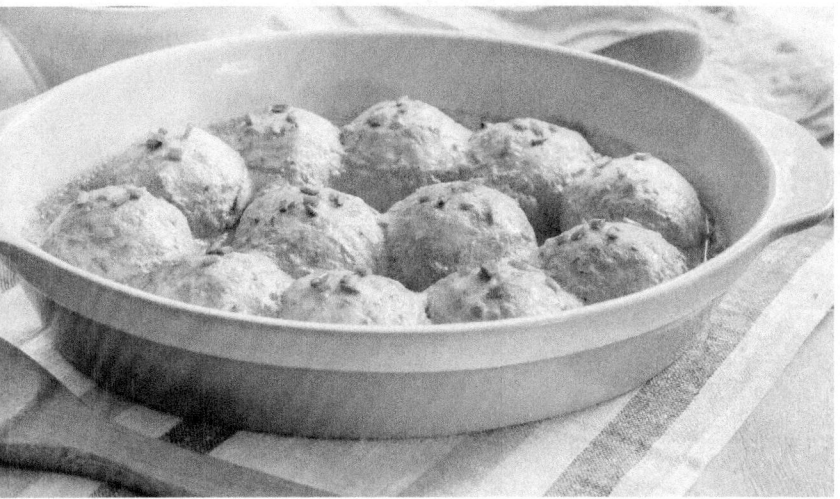

Juicy turkey meatballs are baked and served with a rich cream sauce. This comforting dish is excellent for any meal.

INGREDIENTS

For the Turkey Meatballs:
- 1 lb ground turkey
- Salt, to taste
- Freshly ground black pepper (as much as preferred)
- 1 tablespoon beef tallow or pork lard (for greasing)

For the Cream Sauce:
- 1/2 cup heavy cream
- Salt, to taste
- Freshly ground black pepper (as much as preferred)

NUTRITIONAL INFO

Cal 500 • Fat 40 g • Carb 2 g • Protein 30 g

ALLERGEN INFO

INSTRUCTIONS

1. Commence by preheating your oven to 400°F (200°C).
2. Combine the ground turkey with pepper and salt to taste in a mixing bowl. Mix until well combined.
3. Shape the seasoned turkey mixture into meatballs about 1 inch in diameter.
4. Grease a baking sheet with beef tallow or pork lard to prevent sticking.
5. Place the turkey meatballs on the prepared baking sheet, leaving space between each one.
6. Cook in the oven (preheated) until the meatballs are cooked through and golden brown (for 20-25 minutes).
7. Heat the heavy cream over medium heat in a small saucepan.
8. Season your dish according to your personal taste with pepper and salt. Stir well to combine.
9. Place the meatballs on a serving dish once they are cooked.
10. Pour the warm cream sauce over the meatballs and serve hot.

CHICKEN MEATBALLS
WITH CREAMY CHEESE SAUCE

SERVING 2
PREP TIME: 15 MIN
COOK TIME: 25 MIN

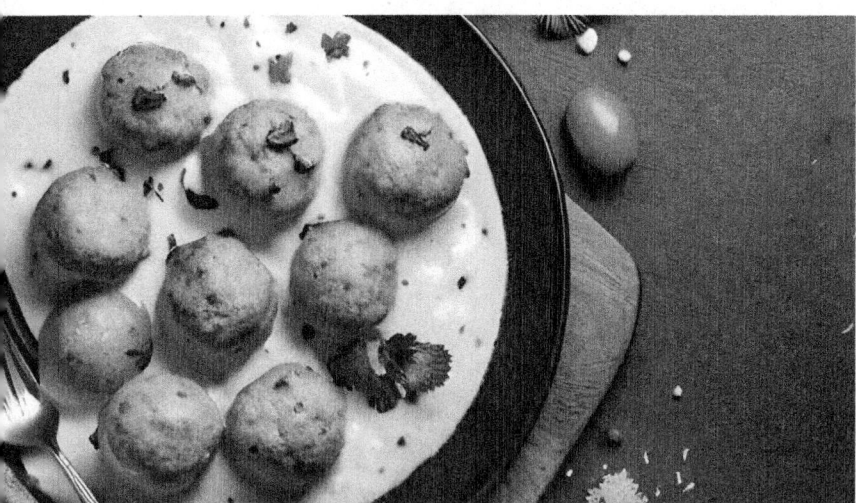

Flavorful chicken meatballs smothered in a creamy cheese sauce—this indulgent dish is sure to please cheese lovers.

INGREDIENTS

For the Chicken Meatballs:
- 1 lb ground chicken
- Salt, to taste
- Freshly ground black pepper (as much as preferred)
- 1 tablespoon beef tallow or pork lard (for greasing)

For the Creamy Cheese Sauce:
- 1/2 cup heavy cream
- 1/4 cup shredded cheddar, mozzarella or other cheese
- Salt, to taste
- Freshly ground black pepper (as much as preferred)

NUTRITIONAL INFO

Cal 550 • Fat 45 g • Carb 0 g • Protein 30 g

ALLERGEN INFO

INSTRUCTIONS

1. Commence by preheating your oven to 400°F (200°C).
2. Blend the ground chicken, adding pepper and salt to taste. Mix until well combined.
3. Shape the seasoned chicken mixture into meatballs about 1 inch in diameter.
4. Grease a baking sheet with beef tallow or pork lard to prevent sticking.
5. Place the chicken meatballs on the prepared baking sheet, leaving space between each one.
6. Cook in the oven (preheated) until the meatballs are cooked through and golden brown (for 20-25 minutes).
7. In a small saucepan, warm the heavy cream until it just begins to simmer (over medium heat).
8. Lower the heat and gently mix the shredded cheese until it melts, making the sauce smooth.
9. Add salt as well as freshly ground black pepper according to your taste preferences. Stir well to combine.
10. Transfer the meatballs to a serving dish once they are cooked.
11. Pour the warm creamy cheese sauce over the meatballs and serve hot.

ROAST GOOSE
WITH SAGE AND THYME

SERVING 2
PREP TIME: 20 MIN
COOK TIME: 3 HOURS

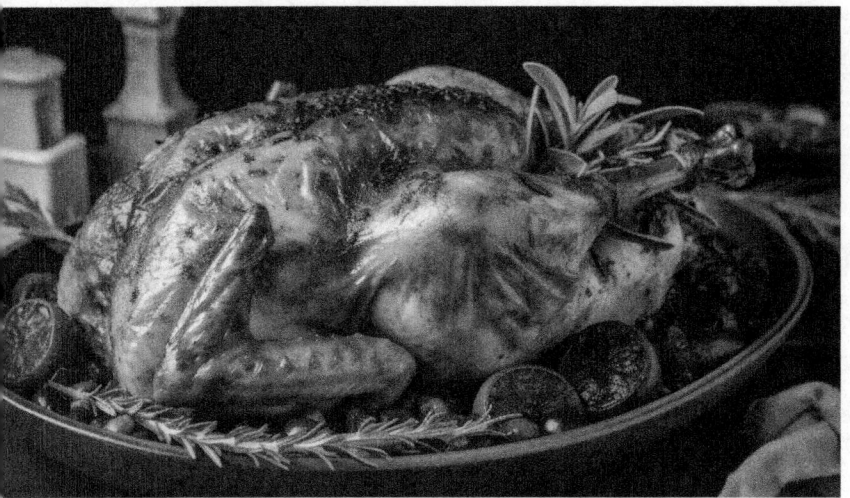

Whole goose roasted with fresh sage and thyme, delivering a festive and hearty main course. Ideal for holiday feasts.

INGREDIENTS

- 1 whole goose, approximately 5-6 pounds
- Salt and black pepper to taste
- 4-6 sprigs fresh sage
- 4-6 sprigs fresh thyme
- 4 cloves garlic, peeled

NUTRITIONAL INFO

Cal 600 • Fat 40 g • Carb 0 g • Protein 50 g

INSTRUCTIONS

1. Commence by preheating your oven to 375°F (190°C).
2. Rinse the goose under cold water and pat dry with paper towels.
3. Season the goose cavity generously with salt and black pepper.
4. Stuff the goose cavity with fresh sage, thyme sprigs, and garlic cloves.
5. Truss the goose with kitchen twine to ensure even cooking.
6. Place the goose on a rack in a roasting pan.
7. Roast the goose for about 2.5 or 3 hours in the preheated oven until the skin is crispy golden brown and the internal temperature is 165°F (75°C) (when measured in the thickest part of the thigh).
8. Baste the goose with its rendered fat and juices every 30 minutes during the cooking process to keep it moist and flavorful.
9. Once cooked, put the goose out of the oven and rest it before carving (for 15-20 minutes).
10. Carve the roasted goose into serving portions and serve hot.

DUCK ROULADE
WITH FRENCH HERBS

SERVING 2
PREP TIME: 20 MIN
COOK TIME: 20 MIN

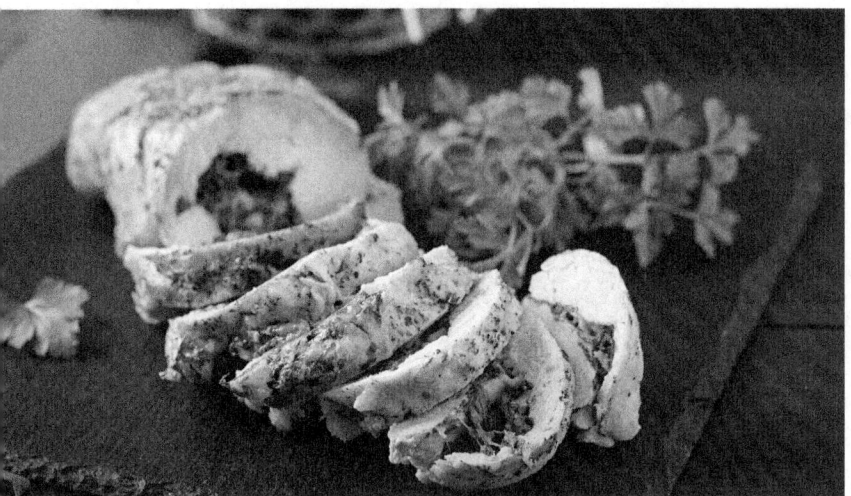

Duck breasts are rolled with prosciutto and fresh herbs and baked to perfection. This dish offers a gourmet twist on poultry.

INGREDIENTS

- 2 duck breasts
- Salt and black pepper to taste
- 2 tablespoons fresh herbs (chopped) like parsley, thyme, and rosemary
- 4 slices prosciutto or bacon
- 2 tablespoons butter or duck fat

NUTRITIONAL INFO

Cal 300 • Fat 25 g • Carb 0 g • Protein 30 g

INSTRUCTIONS

1. Set the temperature in the oven to 375°F or 190°C.
2. Sandwich one duck breast between two plastic wrap sheets. Pound the duck breast using a rolling pin or meat mallet to an equal thickness of about 1/4 inch.
3. Season the mashed duck breast with both black pepper and salt.
4. Evenly distribute half of the chopped fresh herbs throughout the duck breast's surface.
5. Slightly overlap two pieces of prosciutto or bacon on the seared duck breast.
6. Tightly roll up the duck breast, beginning from one end, to form a roulade. Attach the roll firmly with kitchen twine.
7. Proceed with the procedure using the leftover duck breast.
8. Preheat butter or duck fat over medium-high heat in an ovenproof skillet.
9. After the skillet is hot, add the duck rounds and sear them for two to three minutes on each side or until golden brown.
10. Slide the skillet into the warmed oven and bake the duck rolls for fifteen to twenty-five minutes to make sure that the food's internal temperature reaches 165°F (75°C) which means it's cooked.
11. After cooking, remove the duck roasts from the oven and allow them to cool for a few minutes before slicing.
12. Cut the duck rounds into thick rounds after removing the kitchen twine.

CHICKEN CHEESE KEBAB

SERVING 2
PREP TIME: 20 MIN
COOK TIME: 15 MIN

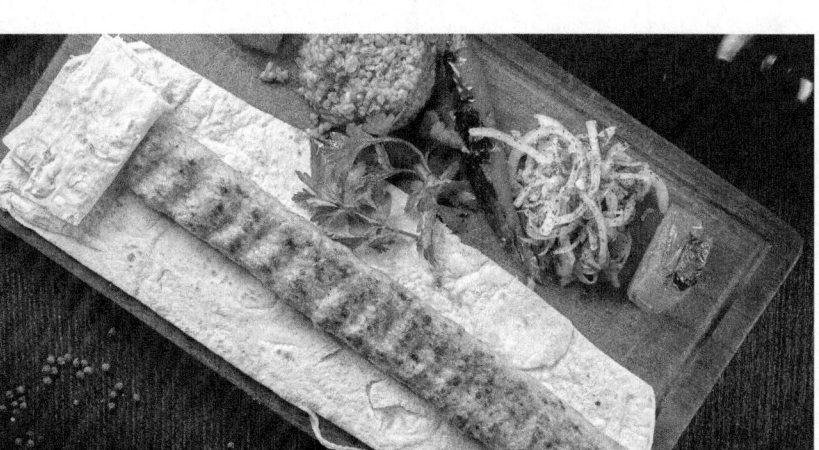

Ground chicken mixed with shredded cheese, shaped into kebabs, and grilled—a tasty and protein-packed option for any meal.

INGREDIENTS

- 1 lb ground chicken
- 1/2 cup shredded mozzarella, cheddar or other cheese
- Salt, to taste
- Freshly ground black pepper (as much as preferred)
- 1 tablespoon beef tallow or pork lard (for greasing)

NUTRITIONAL INFO

Cal 600 • Fat 45 g • Carb 0 g • Protein 45 g

ALLERGEN INFO

INSTRUCTIONS

1. Preheat your grill to medium-high heat.
2. Combine the ground chicken with shredded cheese in a mixing bowl.
3. Add salt as well as freshly ground black pepper to taste.
4. Mix until the cheese is evenly distributed throughout the chicken mixture.
5. Divide the chicken cheese mixture into equal portions and shape each portion into a kebab or sausage shape.
6. Grease the grill grates with beef tallow or pork lard to prevent sticking.
7. Place the chicken cheese kebabs on the preheated grill.
8. Grill 6-8 minutes on each side or until the kebabs are cooked through and have grill marks.
9. Once cooked, remove the chicken cheese kebabs from the grill and place them on a serving platter.
10. Serve hot with your favorite carnivore-friendly dipping sauce, or enjoy them as they are.

CHICKEN FRICASSEE
WITH CREAMY DOR BLUE SAUCE

SERVING 2
PREP TIME: 15 MIN
COOK TIME: 30 MIN

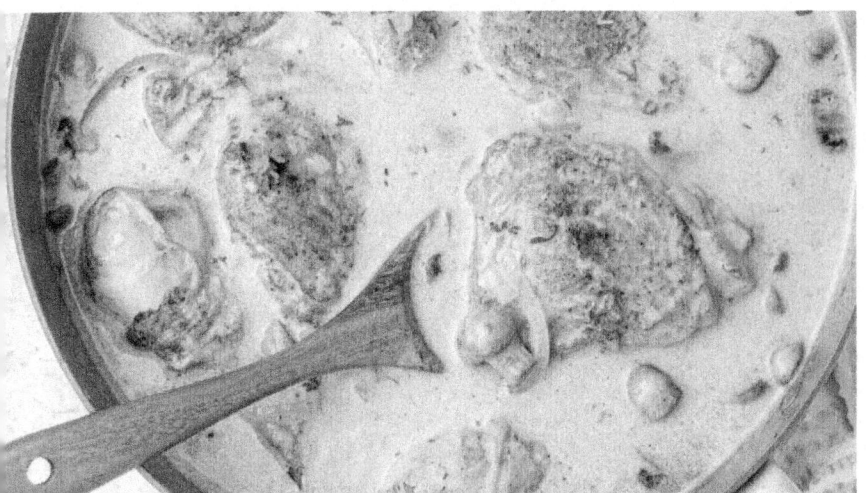

Tender chicken pieces cooked in a creamy blue cheese sauce. This luxurious dish is perfect for a special dinner.

INGREDIENTS

- 2 boneless, skinless chicken breasts
- Salt, to taste
- Freshly ground black pepper (as much as preferred)
- 2 tablespoons beef tallow or pork lard
- 1/2 cup heavy cream
- 1/4 cup blue cheese (such as Dor Blue or Gorgonzola), crumbled

NUTRITIONAL INFO

Cal 700 • Fat 55 g • Carb 2 g • Protein 45 g

ALLERGEN INFO

INSTRUCTIONS

1. Season the chicken breasts, adding salt and freshly ground black pepper to taste.
2. Heat the beef tallow or pork lard over medium-high heat in a skillet.
3. Add the seasoned chicken breasts to the skillet and cook for 6-8 minutes (each side) until they are golden brown and cooked through. Remove from the skillet and set aside.
4. In the same skillet, reduce the heat to medium-low.
5. Add the heavy cream into the skillet and gently simmer it.
6. Add the crumbled blue cheese to the skillet, then stir until it's melted and the sauce is smooth and creamy.
7. Put the cooked chicken breasts back to the skillet, coating them with the creamy Dor Blue sauce.
8. Allow the chicken to simmer in the sauce for a few minutes, ensuring it is heated.
9. Transfer the chicken fricassee with creamy Dor Blue sauce to serving plates once heated.
10. Garnish with freshly chopped parsley or additional crumbled blue cheese, if desired.

SEAFOOD

100	BAKED SALMON SLICES WRAPPED IN BACON
101	SALMON GRILL WITH CAVIAR SAUCE
102	BAKED MACKEREL AND SALMON ROLLS
103	CRISPY BAKED FISH STICKS
104	SQUID STUFFED
105	GRILLED WHOLE TROUT
106	GRILLED LOBSTER TAILS WITH GARLIC BUTTER
107	BAKED MUSSELS WITH CHEESE
108	MUSSELS IN BLUE CHEESE SAUCE
109	SALT-BAKED FISH

BAKED SALMON SLICES
WRAPPED IN BACON

SERVING 2
PREP TIME: 10 MIN
COOK TIME: 20 MIN

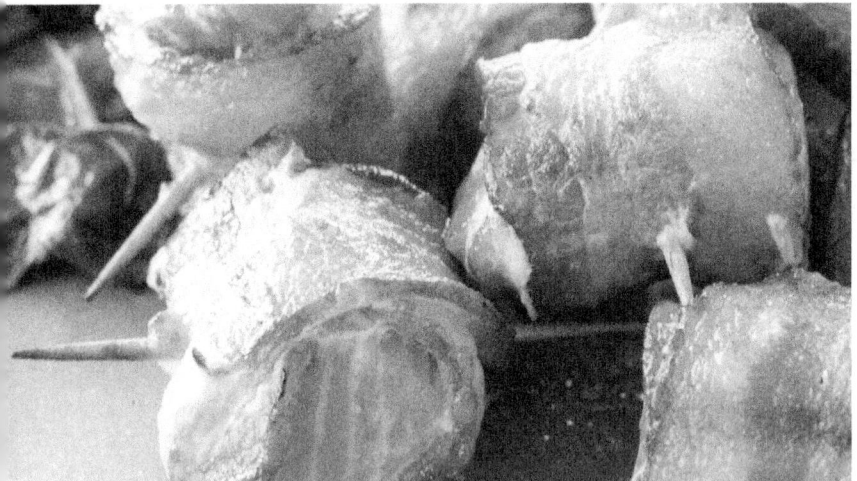

Indulge in the luxurious flavors of salmon slices wrapped in crispy bacon, baked to perfection. This dish combines the rich taste of salmon with the smoky, savory notes of bacon, creating a delightful seafood treat.

INGREDIENTS

- 1/2 lb salmon fillet, cut into 4 slices
- 4 slices of bacon
- Salt, to taste
- Freshly ground black pepper (as much as preferred)

NUTRITIONAL INFO

Cal 600 • Fat 54 g • Carb 0 g • Protein 40 g

ALLERGEN INFO

INSTRUCTIONS

1. Commence by preheating your oven to 400°F (200°C).
2. Season the salmon slices with salt and freshly ground black pepper to taste.
3. Wrap each salmon slice with a slice of bacon. Secure with toothpicks if necessary.
4. Place the bacon-wrapped salmon slices on a tray (covered with parchment paper) or a greased baking sheet.
5. Bake in the oven that has been preheated until the bacon becomes crispy and the salmon is fully cooked(it should take about 15-20 minutes).
6. Once cooked, remove the salmon slices from the oven and let them rest for a few minutes.
7. Serve hot, optionally garnished with a sprig of fresh herbs.

SALMON GRILL
WITH CAVIAR SAUCE

SERVING 2
PREP TIME: 15 MIN
COOK TIME: 10 MIN

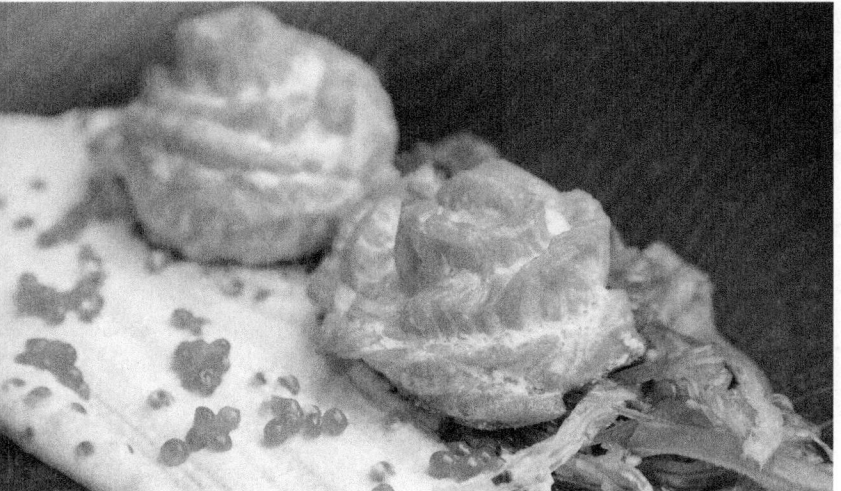

Elevate your seafood experience with grilled salmon topped with a decadent caviar sauce. The combination of tender, juicy salmon and the rich, briny caviar creates a sophisticated dish perfect for special occasions.

INGREDIENTS

For the Grilled Salmon:
- 2 salmon fillets (about 6 oz each)
- Salt, to taste
- Freshly ground black pepper (as much as preferred)
- 1 tablespoon beef tallow or pork lard (for greasing)

For the Caviar Sauce:
- 1/2 cup heavy cream
- 2 tablespoons caviar (such as salmon roe)
- Salt, to taste
- Freshly ground black pepper (as much as preferred)

NUTRITIONAL INFO

Cal 650 • Fat 50 g • Carb 1 g • Protein 45 g

ALLERGEN INFO

INSTRUCTIONS

1. Preheat your grill to medium-high heat.
2. Season the salmon fillets with pepper and salt to taste.
3. Grease the grill grates with beef tallow or pork lard to prevent sticking.
4. Put the salmon fillets on the preheated grill.
5. Grill 4-5 minutes on each side until the salmon is cooked and has grill marks.
6. While the salmon is grilling, heat the heavy cream until it simmers over medium heat.
7. Please reduce the temperature and carefully mix in the caviar.
8. Add salt as well as freshly ground black pepper to taste.
9. Keep the sauce warm on low heat until ready to serve.
10. Once the salmon is cooked, transfer it to serving plates.
11. Spoon the warm caviar sauce over the grilled salmon fillets.

BAKED MACKEREL AND
SALMON ROLLS

SERVING 2
PREP TIME: 15 MIN
COOK TIME: 25 MIN

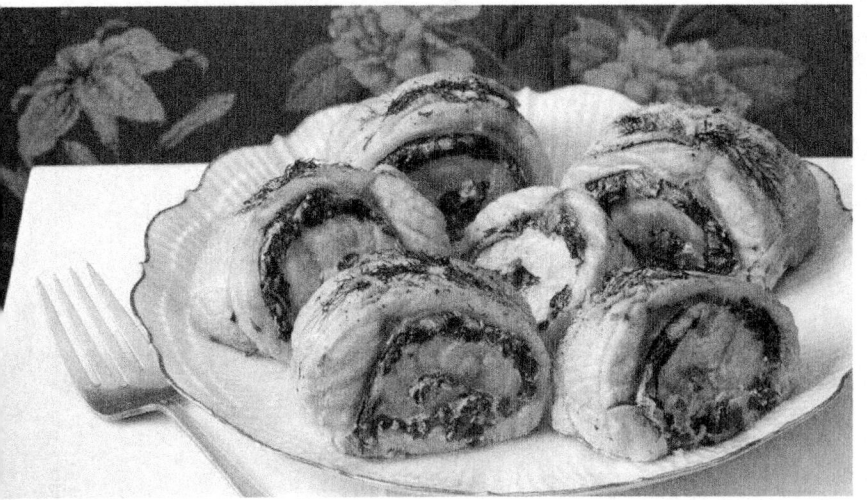

Enjoy the best of both worlds with these baked rolls featuring mackerel and salmon. The blend of these two fish varieties provides a unique and flavorful seafood dish that's both nutritious and delicious.

INGREDIENTS

- 2 mackerel fillets (about 6 oz each)
- 2 salmon fillets (about 6 oz each)
- Salt, to taste
- Freshly ground black pepper (as much as preferred)
- 1 tablespoon beef tallow or pork lard (for greasing)
- Optional: 1 tablespoon fresh herbs (such as dill or parsley), finely chopped

NUTRITIONAL INFO

Cal 700 • Fat 55 g • Carb 0 g • Protein 50 g

ALLERGEN INFO

INSTRUCTIONS

1. Commence by preheating your oven to 375°F (190°C).
2. Season the mackerel and salmon fillets with pepper and salt to taste.
3. If using, sprinkle the fresh herbs evenly over the fillets.
4. Lay each mackerel fillet flat and place a salmon fillet on top.
5. Roll each pair of fillets together tightly and secure with toothpicks if necessary.
6. Grease a beef tallow or pork lard baking dish to prevent sticking.
7. Place the mackerel and salmon rolls in the prepared baking dish.
8. Bake in the oven that has been preheated for 20-25 minutes or until the fish is cooked and can be flaked easily with a fork.
9. Once baked, remove the fish rolls from the oven and let them rest for a few minutes.
10. Serve hot, optionally garnished with additional fresh herbs.

CRISPY BAKED FISH STICKS

SERVING 2
PREP TIME: 10 MIN
COOK TIME: 10 MIN

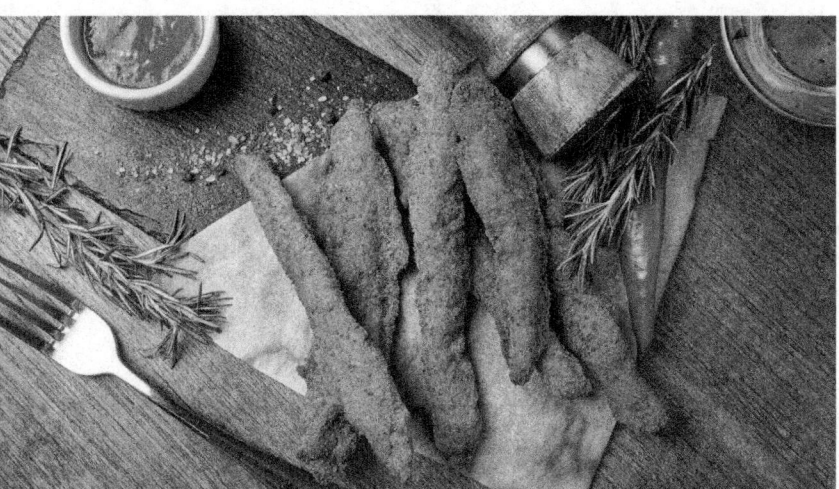

These crispy baked fish sticks are a healthier take on a classic favorite. Made with fresh fish fillets and baked to a golden crisp, they are perfect for a quick and satisfying snack or meal.

INGREDIENTS

- 1 lb cod, haddock, or pollock fillets cut into strips
- 2 eggs, beaten
- 1/2 cup grated Parmesan cheese
- Salt, to taste
- Freshly ground black pepper (as much as preferred)

NUTRITIONAL INFO

Cal 250 • Fat 15 g • Carb 0 g • Protein 27 g

ALLERGEN INFO

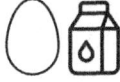

INSTRUCTIONS

1. Commence by preheating your oven to 400°F (200°C).
2. Please be sure to prepare the baking tray (cover it with parchment paper or lightly grease it with beef tallow or pork lard).
3. Season the fish fillet strips with salt and freshly ground black pepper to taste.
4. Place the beaten eggs in one bowl.
5. Place the grated Parmesan cheese in another bowl.
6. Dip each fish strip into the beaten eggs, allowing any excess to drip off.
7. Roll the egg-coated fish strip in the grated Parmesan cheese until well-coated.
8. Place the coated fish strips on the prepared tray for baking, leaving space between each strip.
9. Bake in the oven that has been preheated for about 10 minutes, or until the fish sticks are golden brown and crispy and the fish is cooked through.
10. Once baked, remove the fish sticks from the oven and let them rest for a few minutes.
11. Serve hot, optionally, with a carnivore-friendly dipping sauce.

SQUID STUFFED

SERVING 2
PREP TIME: 15 MIN
COOK TIME: 15 MIN

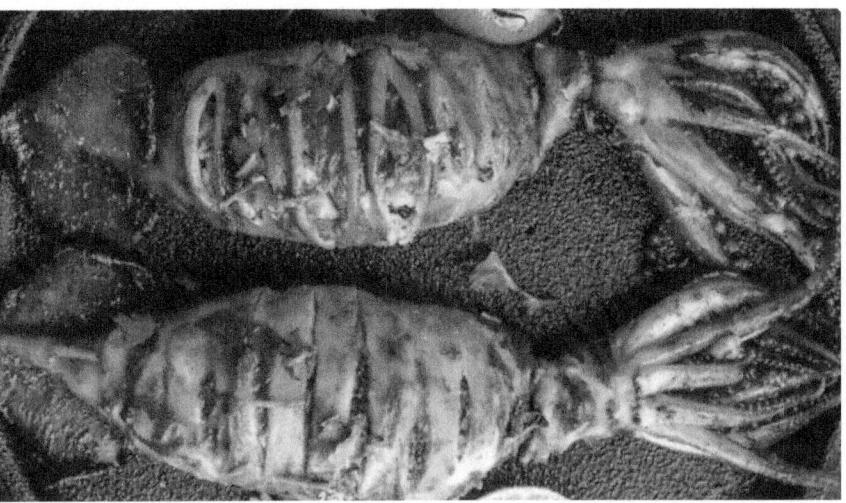

Discover stuffed squid's delicate and savory flavors, filled with a flavorful mixture that enhances its natural taste. This dish is a seafood lover's dream, offering a delightful blend of textures and tastes.

INGREDIENTS

- 2 large squid tubes, cleaned and prepared
- 1/2 lb shrimp, peeled and deveined
- 1/2 lb skinless and boneless breast of a chicken
- Salt, to taste
- Freshly ground black pepper (as much as preferred)
- Cooking fat (such as bacon fat, ghee, or preferred cooking oil)

NUTRITIONAL INFO

Cal 250 • Fat 15 g • Carb 0 g • Protein 35 g

ALLERGEN INFO

INSTRUCTIONS

1. Commence by preheating your oven to 375°F (190°C).
2. Finely chop the shrimp and chicken breast.
3. Mix the chopped shrimp and chicken in a bowl.
4. Add salt as well as freshly ground black pepper to taste.
5. Carefully stuff each squid tube with the shrimp and chicken mixture.
6. Secure the open end of each squid tube with toothpicks to keep the filling inside.
7. Heat your chosen cooking fat over medium-high heat in a skillet.
8. Sear the stuffed squid tubes for 2-3 minutes on each side until lightly browned.
9. Transfer the seared squid tubes to a baking dish.
10. Bake the stuffed squid in the preheated oven for about 10 minutes or until the squid is fully cooked and tender.
11. Once cooked, remove the stuffed squid from the oven and let them rest for a few minutes.
12. Slice the stuffed squid tubes into rounds and serve hot.

GRILLED WHOLE TROUT

> **SERVING 2**
> PREP TIME: 5 MIN
> COOK TIME: 15 MIN

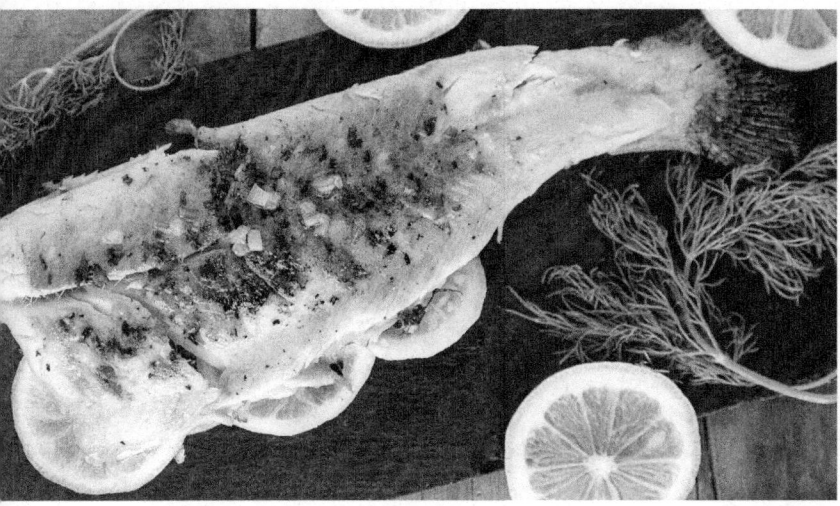

Savor the simplicity and elegance of grilled whole trout, seasoned and perfectly cooked. The fresh, mild trout flavor makes this dish a light and healthy option for any seafood enthusiast.

INGREDIENTS

- 2 whole trout, cleaned and gutted
- Salt, to taste
- Freshly ground black pepper (as much as preferred)
- Cooking fat (such as bacon fat, ghee, or preferred cooking oil)

NUTRITIONAL INFO

Cal 300 • Fat 15 g • Carb 0 g • Protein 30 g

INSTRUCTIONS

1. Preheat your grill to medium-high heat.
2. Season the cleaned and gutted trout inside and out with salt and freshly ground black pepper to taste.
3. Brush the grill grates with your chosen cooking fat to prevent the fish from sticking.
4. Place the trout on the preheated grill.
5. Cook the fish on the grill for 7-8 minutes on each side until the skin becomes crispy and the fish is cooked so that it can be flaked easily with a fork.
6. Once cooked, carefully remove the trout from the grill.
7. Let the fish rest for a few minutes before serving.

GRILLED LOBSTER TAILS
WITH GARLIC BUTTER

SERVING 2
PREP TIME: 10 MIN
COOK TIME: 10 MIN

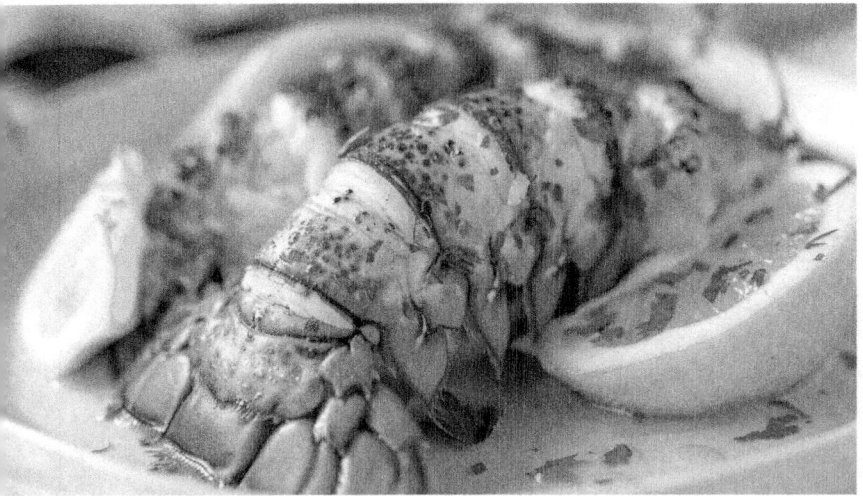

Treat yourself to the luxurious taste of grilled lobster tails drizzled with rich garlic butter. The tender lobster meat and the savory butter sauce create an indulgent and unforgettable dish.

INGREDIENTS

- 2 lobster tails, thawed if frozen
- 4 tablespoons unsalted butter, melted
- 2 cloves garlic, minced
- Salt, to taste
- Freshly ground black pepper (as much as preferred)
- Lemon wedges for serving (optional)

NUTRITIONAL INFO

Cal 250 • Fat 20 g • Carb 2 g • Protein 25 g

ALLERGEN INFO

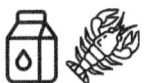

INSTRUCTIONS

1. Preheat your grill to medium-high heat.
2. Use kitchen shears to cut down the top shell of each lobster tail, stopping at the base of the tail.
3. Pull apart the shell and lift the lobster meat slightly, resting it on top of the shell.
4. Mix the melted butter and minced garlic in a bowl.
5. Brush the lobster meat generously with the garlic butter.
6. Add salt as well as freshly ground black pepper to taste.
7. Place the lobster tails, meat side up, on the preheated grill.
8. Grill for about 5-6 minutes, then turn and grill for another 4-5 minutes or until the meat is opaque and cooked through.
9. Once cooked, remove the lobster tails from the grill.
10. Serve hot, optionally, with lemon wedges on the side.

BAKED MUSSELS
WITH CHEESE

SERVING 2
PREP TIME: 15 MIN
COOK TIME: 15 MIN

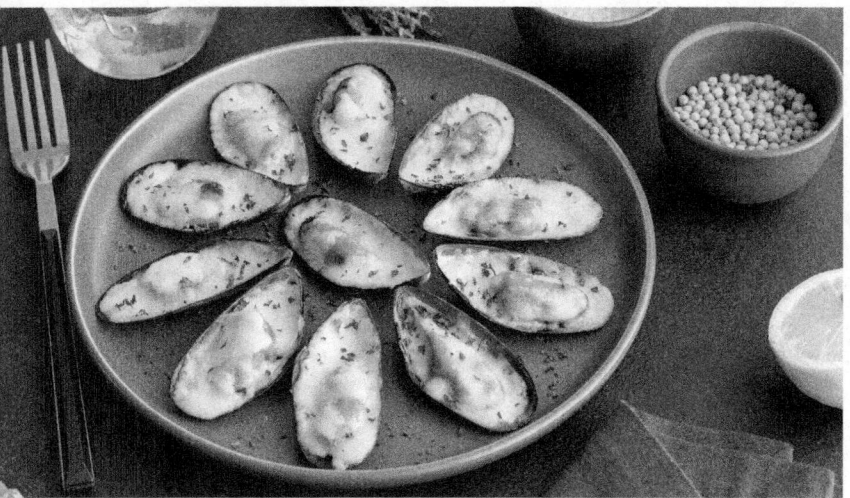

These baked mussels are topped with a savory cheese blend and baked until bubbly and golden. This delightful appetizer or main course showcases the rich flavors of fresh mussels.

INGREDIENTS

- 2 lbs fresh mussels, cleaned and debearded
- 1/2 cup grated Parmesan or Gruyère cheese
- 2 tablespoons butter, melted
- Salt and black pepper to taste

NUTRITIONAL INFO

Cal 350 • Fat 25 g • Carb 2g • Protein 35 g

ALLERGEN INFO

 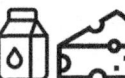

INSTRUCTIONS

1. Commence by preheating your oven to 400°F (200°C).
2. Arrange the cleaned mussels in a single layer in a baking dish.
3. In a small bowl, mix the grated cheese, melted butter, salt, and black pepper.
4. Spoon the cheese mixture over each mussel, dividing it evenly among them.
5. Put the dish for baking into the oven that has been preheated and cook until the cheese is bubbly and melted and the mussels are cooked through (for 12-15 minutes).
6. Once baked, remove the baking dish from the oven and let it cool for a few minutes.

MUSSELS IN BLUE
CHEESE SAUCE

SERVING 2
PREP TIME: 10 MIN
COOK TIME: 10 MIN

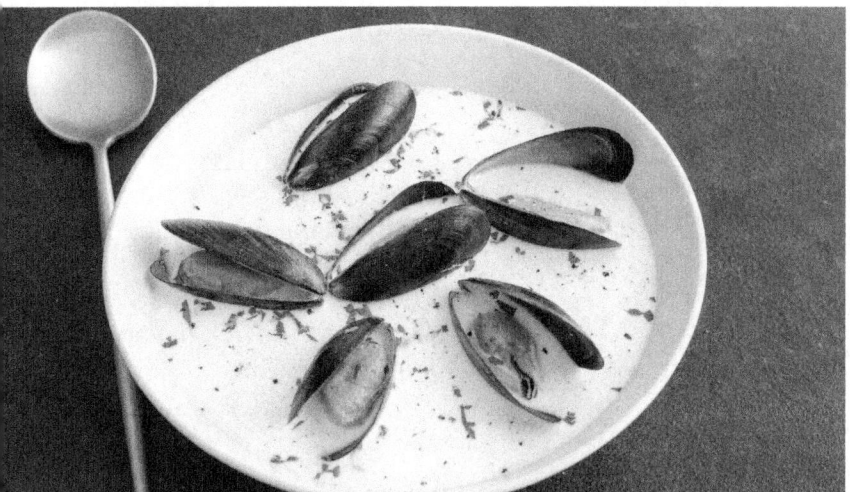

Experience mussels' bold and creamy flavors cooked in a luscious blue cheese sauce. The tangy blue cheese complements the briny mussels, creating a unique and flavorful seafood dish.

INGREDIENTS

- 2 lbs fresh mussels, cleaned and debearded
- 1 cup broth (chicken or vegetable)
- 1/2 cup blue cheese, crumbled
- Salt and black pepper to taste
- Chopped fresh parsley for garnish (optional)

INSTRUCTIONS

1. Bring the broth to a pot to a simmer over medium heat.
2. Add the cleaned mussels to the pot and cover with a lid. Cook for about 5-7 minutes or until the mussels have opened up.
3. While the mussels are cooking, crumble the blue cheese into a small saucepan and melt it over low heat, stirring occasionally.
4. Once the mussels have opened, use a slotted spoon to place them on a serving bowl, discarding unopened ones.
5. Pour the melted blue cheese sauce over the cooked mussels.
6. Season with pepper and salt to taste.

NUTRITIONAL INFO

Cal 400 • Fat 20 g • Carb 2g • Protein 45 g

ALLERGEN INFO

SALT-BAKED FISH

> **SERVING 2**
> PREP TIME: 15 MIN
> COOK TIME: 35 MIN

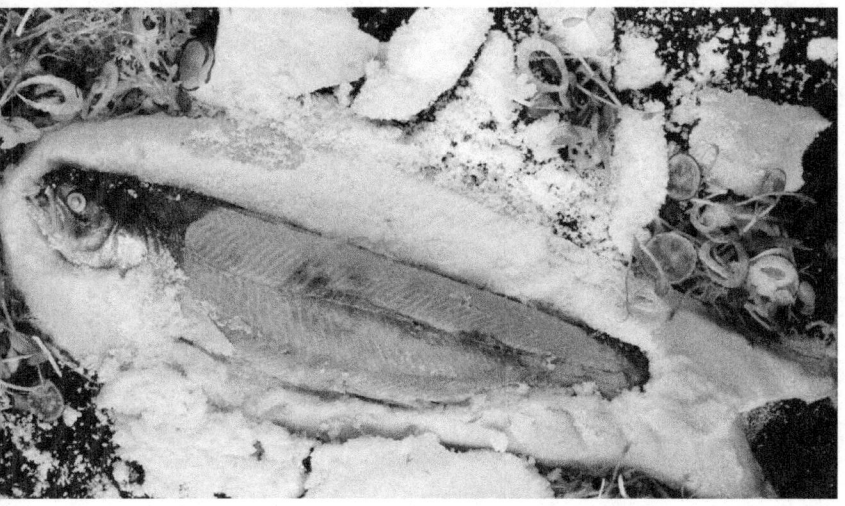

Enjoy the tender, flavorful meat of salt-baked fish cooked to perfection under a sea salt crust. This cooking method locks in moisture and enhances the fish's natural flavors, making it a simple yet exquisite dish.

INGREDIENTS

- 2 whole fish (such as sea bass, trout, or snapper), cleaned and scaled
- 4 cups coarse sea salt
- 2 egg whites
- Fresh thyme, rosemary, or dill for stuffing

NUTRITIONAL INFO

Cal 250 • Fat 15 g • Carb 0g • Protein 35 g

INSTRUCTIONS

1. Commence by preheating your oven to 400°F (200°C).
2. Combine the coarse sea salt and egg whites in a mixing bowl. Mix well until the salt is evenly moistened and holds together when squeezed.
3. Stuff the cavities of the cleaned and scaled whole fish with fresh herbs and lemon slices.
4. Spread a layer of the salt mixture in the bottom of a baking dish or roasting pan.
5. Place the stuffed whole fish on top of the salt layer.
6. Cover the fish with the remaining salt mixture, pressing it gently to form a thick crust around it.
7. Transfer the baking dish or roasting pan to the oven that has been preheated and bake for 30-40 mins (depending on the fish size) until the salt crust is golden brown and hardened.
8. Once baked, remove the salt-crusted fish from the oven and let it rest for a few minutes.
9. Carefully crack open the salt crust using a spoon or knife and remove it from the fish.
10. Gently brush off any excess salt from the surface of the fish.

OFFAL

111 CHICKEN HEARTS IN SOUR CREAM
112 CHICKEN LIVER IN CURRY CREAM SAUCE
113 CHICKEN LIVER PÂTÉ
114 BEEF TONGUE ASPIC
115 BOILED BEEF TONGUE ROLLS STUFFED
116 LIVER, TONGUE, AND EGGS SKILLET
117 LIVER PANCAKES
118 LAMB BRAIN SCRAMBLE
119 CHICKEN GIBLET GRAVY
120 HOMEMADE TONGUE, LIVER, AND HEART SAUSAGES

CHICKEN HEARTS
IN SOUR CREAM

SERVING 2
PREP TIME: 10 MIN
COOK TIME: 20 MIN

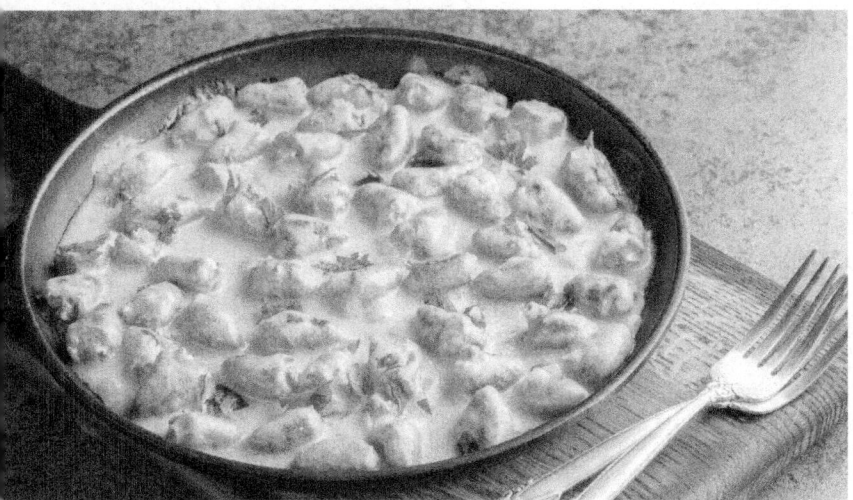

Savor the rich and creamy flavor of tender chicken hearts cooked perfectly in a luscious sour cream sauce. This dish offers a delightful combination of texture and taste, perfect for a gourmet carnivore experience.

INGREDIENTS

- 1 lb chicken hearts, cleaned
- 2 tablespoons beef tallow or ghee (for cooking)
- 1 cup sour cream
- Salt, to taste
- Freshly ground black pepper (as much as preferred)

NUTRITIONAL INFO

Cal 350 • Fat 25 g • Carb 2g • Protein 30 g

ALLERGEN INFO

INSTRUCTIONS

1. Clean the chicken hearts by trimming excess fat and connective tissue.
2. In a skillet, heat the beef tallow or ghee over medium-high heat.
3. Add the cleaned chicken hearts to the skillet.
4. Add salt as well as freshly ground black pepper to taste.
5. Cook, stirring occasionally, until the hearts are browned on all sides, about 8-10 minutes.
6. At this point, lower the heat to medium and incorporate the sour cream into the mixture.
7. Ensure the hearts are evenly coated with the sour cream.
8. Simmer for an additional 10 minutes, allowing the sauce to thicken and the hearts to cook through.
9. Once cooked, remove the dish from heat and rest for a few minutes.
10. Serve hot, garnished with additional freshly ground black pepper if desired.

CHICKEN LIVER IN CURRY
CREAM SAUCE

> **SERVING 2**
> PREP TIME: 10 MIN
> COOK TIME: 20 MIN

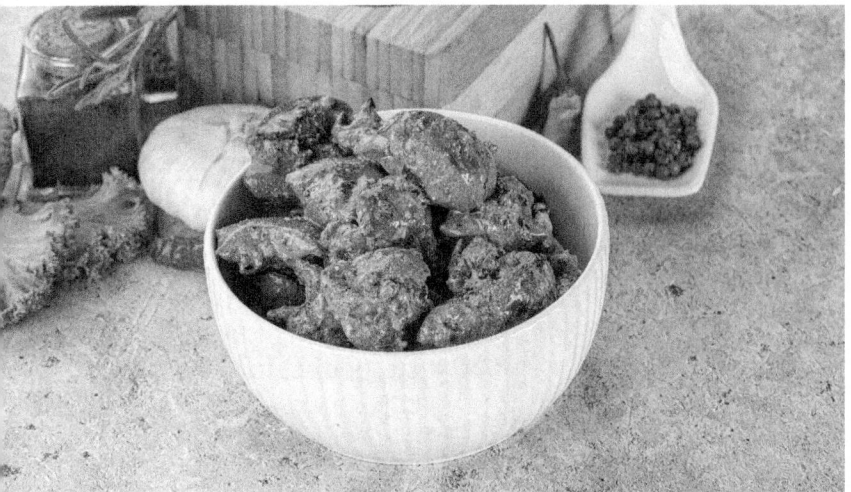

Experience a bold fusion of flavors with this exotic dish, which simmers chicken livers in a savory curry cream sauce. It's a delightful way to enjoy nutrient-rich offal with a spicy twist.

INGREDIENTS

- 1 lb chicken liver, cleaned and trimmed
- 2 tablespoons beef tallow or ghee (for cooking)
- 1 cup heavy cream
- 1 tablespoon curry powder
- Salt, to taste
- Freshly ground black pepper (as much as preferred)

NUTRITIONAL INFO

Cal 400 • Fat 30 g • Carb 4g • Protein 28 g

ALLERGEN INFO

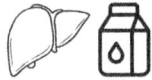

INSTRUCTIONS

1. Clean and trim the chicken livers by removing connective tissue and cutting them into uniform pieces.
2. Heat the beef tallow or ghee over medium-high heat in a skillet.
3. Put the chicken livers in the skillet.
4. Add salt as well as freshly ground black pepper to taste.
5. Cook, stirring occasionally, until the livers are browned on all sides, about 5-7 minutes.
6. Sprinkle the curry powder over the browned livers.
7. Stir well to coat the livers evenly with the curry powder.
8. Reduce the heat to medium and stir in the heavy cream.
9. Ensure the livers are evenly coated with the cream.
10. Simmer for 10-12 minutes, allowing the sauce to thicken and the livers to cook through.
11. Once cooked, remove the dish from heat and rest for a few minutes.
12. Serve hot, garnished with additional freshly ground black pepper if desired.

CHICKEN LIVER PÂTÉ

SERVING 2
PREP TIME: 10 MIN
COOK TIME: 15 MIN

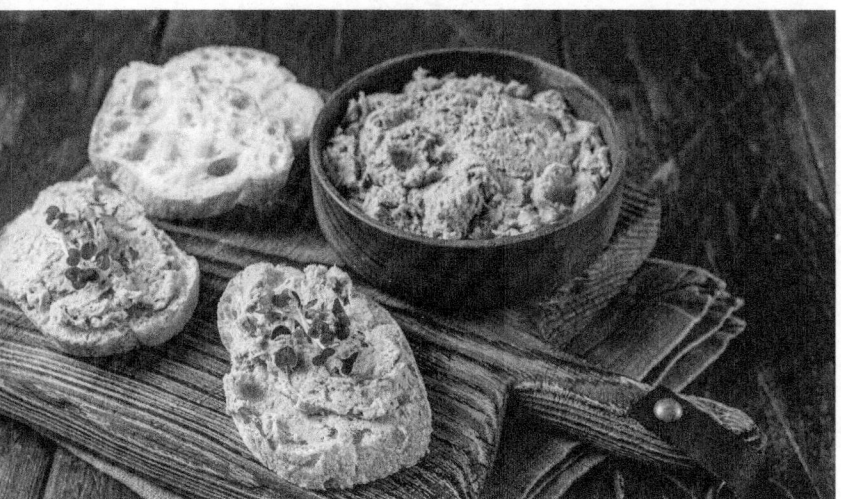

Experience the velvety and opulent consistency of this timeless chicken liver pâté, elevated with gentle spices for a sophisticated starter. Perfect for spreading on your favorite carnivore-friendly crackers.

INGREDIENTS

- 1 lb chicken liver, cleaned
- 1/2 cup heavy cream
- Salt, to taste
- Freshly ground black pepper (as much as preferred)
- Optional: butter (for sealing)

NUTRITIONAL INFO

Cal 300 • Fat 25 g • Carb 2g • Protein 15 g

ALLERGEN INFO

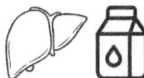

INSTRUCTIONS

1. Heat some beef tallow or ghee over medium-high heat in a skillet.
2. Add the cleaned chicken livers to the skillet and add salt as well as freshly ground black pepper to taste.
3. Fry them up until the livers are browned on the outside but still slightly pink on the inside, about 5-7 minutes.
4. Transfer the cooked chicken livers to a food processor.
5. Add the heavy cream to the food processor.
6. Blend until smooth and creamy, scraping down the sides of the processor as needed.
7. Taste the pâté and adjust the seasoning, adding salt or pepper if you want.
8. Transfer the pâté to a serving dish or small ramekins.
9. If desired, melt some butter and pour it over the pâté to create a seal.
10. Wrap the dish or ramekins with plastic wrap, placing it in the refrigerator for a minimum of 2 hours, or until the pâté has set and become firm.

BEEF TONGUE ASPIC

> **SERVING 2**
> PREP TIME: 10 MIN
> COOK TIME: 3 HOURS

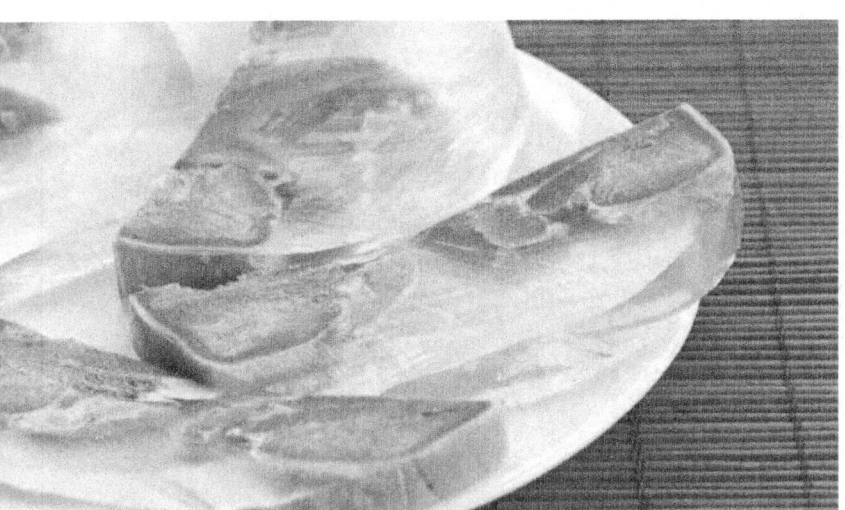

Enjoy a traditional delicacy with beef tongue aspic, where tender slices of beef tongue are encased in savory gelatin. This dish is visually stunning and rich in flavor, making it a perfect centerpiece.

INGREDIENTS

- 1 beef tongue (about 1 lb), cleaned
- 4 cups beef broth
- 1 packet of unflavored gelatin (about 7 g)
- Salt, to taste
- Freshly ground black pepper (as much as preferred)

NUTRITIONAL INFO

Cal 400 • Fat 30 g • Carb 0g • Protein 35 g

INSTRUCTIONS

1. Rinse the beef tongue under cold water and pat it dry with paper towels.
2. Cover the beef tongue in a large pot with cold water.
3. Reduce the heat to low when the water boils and simmer for about 2-3 hours or until the tongue is tender. You can also use a pressure cooker for faster cooking.
4. Once the beef tongue is cooked, remove it from the pot and let it cool slightly.
5. Peel off the tough outer skin from the tongue and discard.
6. Slice the cooked tongue into thin slices and place them in a serving dish or individual molds.
7. Pour 1 cup of beef broth into a small saucepan and sprinkle the gelatin over the surface.
8. Let the gelatin soften for a few minutes.
9. Place the saucepan over low heat and stir until the gelatin is completely dissolved.
10. Stir in the remaining beef broth (after removing from the heat) —season with pepper and salt to taste.
11. Carefully pour the gelatin mixture over the sliced beef tongue in the serving dish or molds.
12. Ensure the gelatin mixture fully covers the beef tongue slices.
13. Cover the dish or molds with plastic wrap, placing it into the refrigerator for at least 6 hours or until the gelatin is set and firm.
14. Serve the beef tongue aspic cold as an appetizer or a main dish.

BOILED BEEF TONGUE
ROLLS STUFFED

SERVING 2
PREP TIME: 20 MIN
COOK TIME: 2 HOURS

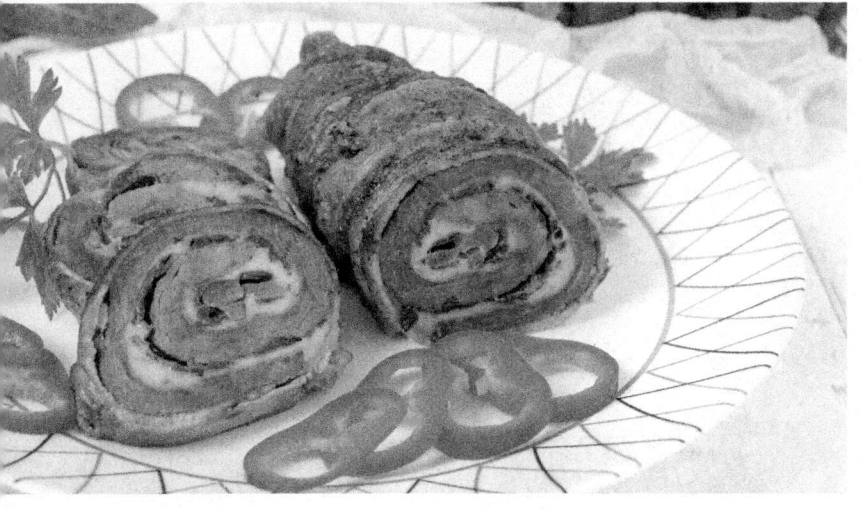

Delight in these flavorful rolls of boiled beef tongue stuffed with a delicious filling that complements the tender meat. This dish is substantial and fulfilling, making it an ideal choice for any meat lover's gathering.

INGREDIENTS

- 1 beef tongue (about 1 lb), cleaned
- 4 cups beef broth
- 1 cup shredded cheddar or mozzarella cheese
- 1/2 cup carnivore mayonnaise
- Salt, to taste
- Freshly ground black pepper (as much as preferred)

NUTRITIONAL INFO

Cal 370 • Fat 30 g • Carb 2g • Protein 30 g

ALLERGEN INFO

INSTRUCTIONS

1. Rinse the beef tongue under cold water and pat it dry with paper towels.
2. Cover the beef tongue in a large pot with beef broth.
3. Reduce the heat to low after bringing the broth to a boil and simmer for about 2 hours or until the tongue is tender.
4. Once the beef tongue is cooked, remove it from the broth and let it cool slightly.
5. Peel off the tough outer skin from the tongue and discard.
6. Slice the cooked tongue into thin slices.
7. Mix the shredded cheese with carnivore mayonnaise in a small bowl until well combined.
8. Season with pepper and salt to taste.
9. Lay out the beef tongue slices on a clean work surface.
10. Spread a small amount of the cheese and mayonnaise filling on one end of each beef tongue slice.
11. Roll up the beef tongue slices, enclosing the filling inside each roll.
12. If needed, use toothpicks to secure the rolls closed.
13. Garnish the beef tongue rolls with chopped fresh herbs if desired.
14. Serve the rolls warm or at room temperature.

LIVER, TONGUE, AND
EGGS SKILLET

SERVING 2
PREP TIME: 10 MIN
COOK TIME: 2 HOURS

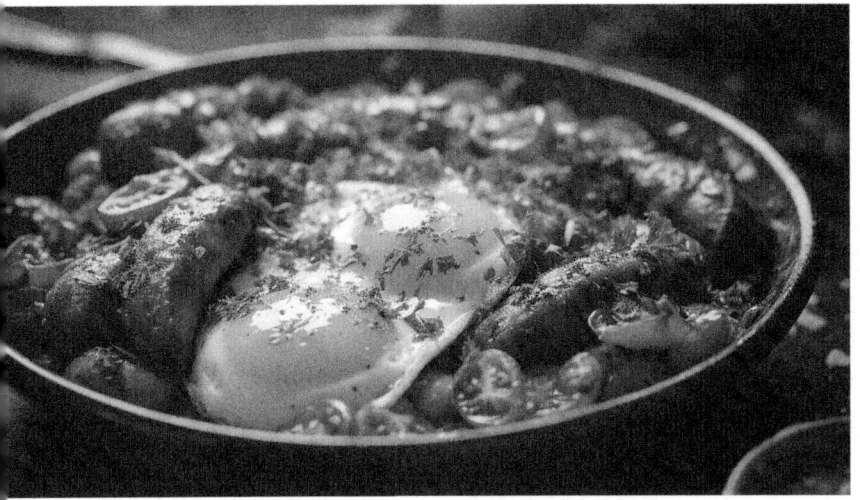

This skillet dish combines the rich flavors of liver, tongue, and eggs, creating a protein-packed meal that's both nutritious and delicious. Perfect for a hearty breakfast or brunch.

INGREDIENTS

- 1 beef tongue (about 1 lb), cleaned
- 1 lb beef liver, sliced
- 4 eggs
- 2 tablespoons beef tallow or ghee
- Salt, to taste
- Freshly ground black pepper (as much as preferred)

NUTRITIONAL INFO

Cal 450 • Fat 35 g • Carb 2g • Protein 30 g

ALLERGEN INFO

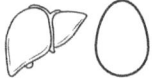

INSTRUCTIONS

1. Rinse the beef tongue under cold water and pat it dry with paper towels.
2. Place the beef tongue in a large pot and cover it with water.
3. Reduce the heat to low after bringing the water to a boil and simmer for about 2 hours or until the tongue is tender.
4. Once the tongue is cooked, remove it from the pot and let it cool slightly. Peel off the tongue's outer skin and discard. Slice the tongue into thin slices.
5. Raise the heat of a skillet (over medium-high heat) and add the beef tallow or ghee. Add the sliced liver to the skillet and cook for 3-4 minutes on each side or until cooked through.
6. Crack the eggs into the pan.
7. Cook the eggs to your desired level of doneness, either sunny-side up, over easy, or scrambled.
8. Once the liver and eggs are cooked, add the sliced beef tongue to the skillet.
9. Season everything with salt and freshly ground black pepper to taste.
10. Gently mix everything in the skillet and keep on cooking for an extra 1-2 minutes to ensure that the dish is heated through.
11. Serve hot directly from the skillet.

LIVER PANCAKES

SERVING 2
PREP TIME: 10 MIN
COOK TIME: 15 MIN

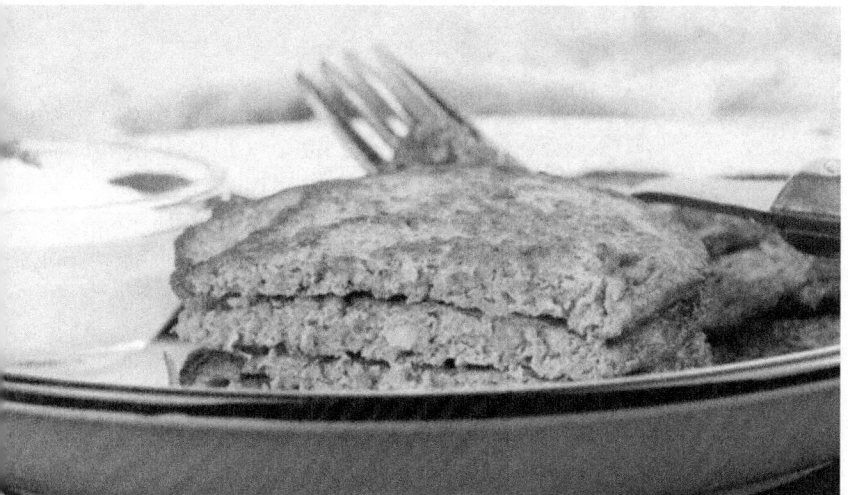

These savory liver pancakes are a unique and delicious method to reap the nutritional advantages of the liver. They're light, fluffy, and perfect for a carnivore-friendly breakfast or snack.

INGREDIENTS

- 1 lb beef liver, cleaned and chopped
- 2 eggs
- 2 tablespoons beef tallow or ghee
- Salt, to taste
- Freshly ground black pepper (as much as preferred)

NUTRITIONAL INFO

Cal 300 • Fat 20 g • Carb 2g • Protein 25 g

ALLERGEN INFO

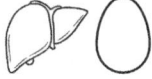

INSTRUCTIONS

1. Rinse the beef liver under cold water and pat it dry with paper towels. Chop it into small pieces.
2. Combine the chopped liver and eggs in a blender or food processor. Blend until you get a smooth mixture.
3. Season the liver mixture with salt and freshly ground black pepper to taste.
4. Proceed by heating a skillet over medium heat, then add the beef tallow or ghee.
5. Once the skillet is hot, pour some of the liver mixture onto the skillet to form small pancakes.
6. Cook the pancakes for about 3-4 minutes on each side or until golden brown and cooked through.
7. Once cooked, remove the liver pancakes from the skillet and place them on a serving plate.
8. Serve hot as they are or with your favorite carnivore-friendly sauce or condiment.

LAMB BRAIN SCRAMBLE

SERVING 2
PREP TIME: 5 MIN
COOK TIME: 10 MIN

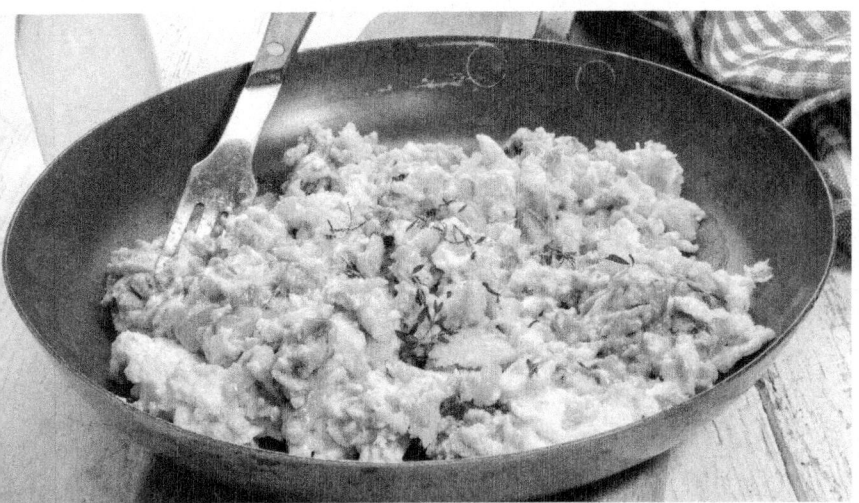

Discover the creamy and delicate flavor of lamb brain in this delightful scramble, perfect for an adventurous breakfast. It's a nutrient-dense dish that brings a gourmet touch to your carnivore diet.

INGREDIENTS

- 8 oz lamb brains (about 2 lamb brains)
- 4 large eggs
- 2 tablespoons beef tallow or ghee
- Salt, to taste
- Freshly ground black pepper (as much as preferred)

NUTRITIONAL INFO

Cal 320 • Fat 25 g • Carb 0 g • Protein 20g

ALLERGEN INFO

INSTRUCTIONS

1. Rinse the lamb brains under cold water and pat them dry with paper towels. Remove any membranes or excess tissue.
2. Proceed by heating a skillet over medium heat, and then add the beef tallow or ghee.
3. Once the skillet is heating hot, add the lamb brains and cook for about 3-4 minutes on each side or until they are lightly browned and cooked through.
4. While the lamb brains cook, crack the eggs, whisking them together in the bowl until well beaten.
5. Once the lamb brains are cooked, remove them from the skillet and chop them into small pieces.
6. Put the skillet back to the heat and add the beaten eggs.
7. Cook the eggs, stirring constantly, until they are scrambled and just set.
8. Add the chopped lamb brains to the skillet once the eggs are cooked.
9. Stir to combine and heat through.
10. Season the lamb brain scramble with salt and freshly ground black pepper to taste.
11. Serve hot directly from the skillet.

CHICKEN GIBLET GRAVY

SERVING 2
PREP TIME: 10 MIN
COOK TIME: 20 MIN

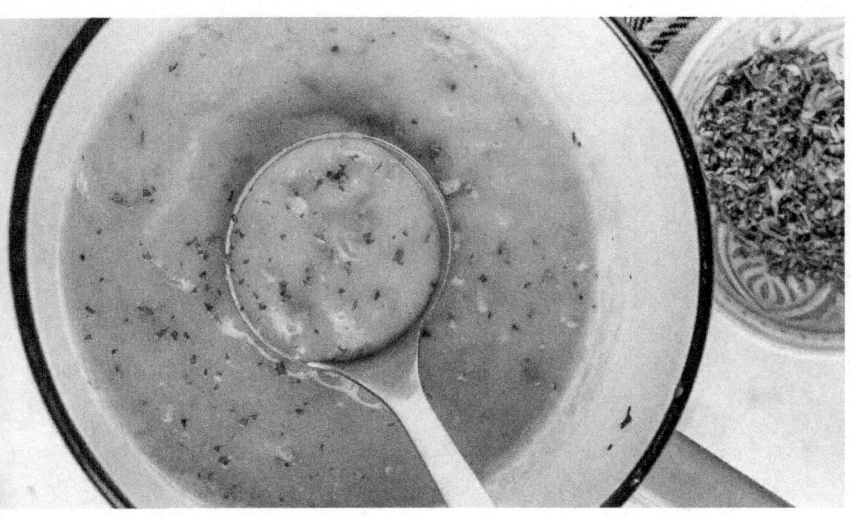

Enhance your meals with this rich and flavorful chicken giblet gravy made from the nutrient-packed organs of the bird. It's perfect for drizzling over your favorite carnivore dishes for an extra flavor boost.

INGREDIENTS

- 1 cup chicken giblets (liver, heart, gizzard), chopped
- 2 cups beef broth
- 2 tablespoons beef tallow or ghee
- Salt, to taste
- Freshly ground black pepper (as much as preferred)

NUTRITIONAL INFO

Cal 180 • Fat 12 g • Carb 0g • Protein 18 g

INSTRUCTIONS

1. Rinse the chicken giblets under cold water and pat them dry with paper towels. Chop them into small pieces.
2. Proceed by heating a skillet over medium heat, and then add the beef tallow or ghee.
3. Once the skillet is heating hot, add the chopped chicken giblets and cook for about 5-7 minutes until they are browned (stir occasionally).
4. Once the giblets are browned, pour the beef broth into the skillet.
5. Stir to combine, scraping up any browned bits from the bottom of the skillet.
6. Bring the mixture to a simmer and let it cook for 10-15 minutes, or until the giblets are cooked through and the gravy thickens to your desired consistency.
7. Season the gravy with salt and freshly ground black pepper to taste.
8. Once the gravy is ready, remove it from the heat.
9. Serve hot over your favorite carnivore-friendly dishes such as roasted or grilled meats.

HOMEMADE TONGUE, LIVER,
AND HEART SAUSAGES

SERVING 2
PREP TIME: 20 MIN
COOK TIME: 20 MIN

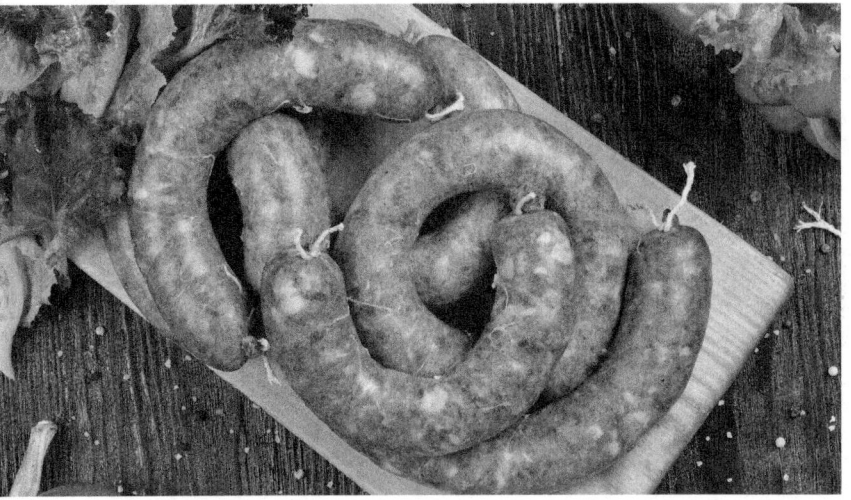

Enjoy these homemade sausages made from a mix of tongue, liver, and heart, offering a blend of rich flavors and textures. They're perfect for a nutritious and satisfying meal any time of the day.

INGREDIENTS

- 8 oz beef tongue, cooked and finely chopped
- 8 oz beef liver, cooked and finely chopped
- 8 oz beef heart, cooked and finely chopped
- 1 egg
- 2 tablespoons beef tallow or ghee
- Salt, to taste
- Freshly ground black pepper (as much as preferred)
- Optional: herbs and spices of your choice

NUTRITIONAL INFO

Cal 280 • Fat 20 g • Carb 0g • Protein 22 g

ALLERGEN INFO

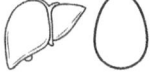

INSTRUCTIONS

1. Cook and cool the beef tongue, liver, and heart before chopping them into fine pieces.
2. Combine the chopped beef tongue, liver, and heart in a mixing bowl.
3. Toss the egg into the mixture and mix well to combine. This will help bind the sausages together.
4. Season the mixture with salt, freshly ground black pepper, and any optional herbs or spices you choose. Mix until evenly distributed.
5. Divide the mix into uniform portions and form each into sausage-shaped patties.
6. Proceed by heating a skillet over medium heat, and then add the beef tallow or ghee.
7. When the skillet becomes hot, add the sausages and cook for about 8-10 minutes on each side or until they are browned and cooked through.
8. Once the sausages are cooked, take them out and let them drain on paper towels to get rid of any extra fat.
9. Serve it while it's hot, either as the main dish or as part of a meal that's carnivore-friendly.

CONCLUSION

EMBRACE YOUR CARNIVORE INSTINCT

As you reach the final pages of "The Carnivore Instinct. Cookbook for Beginners," you've taken the first crucial steps on a journey that reconnects you with the primal, nutrient-dense foods that have sustained humans for millennia. You've explored a diverse range of recipes, each one a celebration of the rich flavors and health benefits that a meat-based diet can offer.

This cookbook isn't just a collection of recipes—it's a guide to transforming your relationship with food, your body, and your health. Whether you came here to lose weight, gain energy, heal naturally, or simply enjoy the unparalleled taste of high-quality meats, you've found a powerful ally in the carnivore lifestyle.

Remember, this is just the beginning. The knowledge and recipes within these pages are tools to help you thrive, but the true power lies in your commitment and willingness to explore this way of eating fully. As you continue on your carnivorous journey, let each meal be a reminder of your connection to nature, your body's needs, and the endless possibilities that come with embracing a diet rich in animal-based nutrition.

So, light the grill, sharpen your knives, and step confidently into a world where meat is more than just food—it's a pathway to optimal health, boundless energy, and a life lived to its fullest potential. Your carnivore instinct is calling—embrace it.

NUTRIENT PROFILES OF ANIMAL-BASED FOODS PER 100 GRAMS

Ingredient	Calories (kcal)	Protein (g)	Fats (g)	Saturated Fats (g)	Carbs (g)	Vitamins	Minerals	Cholesterol (mg)	Sodium (mg)	Omega-3 (g)	Omega-6 (g)
MEATS:											
Beef Bone Marrow	230	7	22	12	0	A, D, E, K2	Calcium, Phosphorus, Magnesium	110	10	0.05	0.1
Beef Brisket	250	27	18	7	0	B1, B2, B3, B5, B6, B12	Iron, Zinc, Selenium	95	75	0.1	0.15
Beef Chuck	275	23	21	9	0	B1, B2, B3, B5, B6, B12	Iron, Zinc, Selenium	105	70	0.1	0.15
Beef Flank	210	21	17	6	0	B1, B2, B3, B5, B6, B12	Iron, Zinc, Selenium	90	65	0.1	0.15
Beef Heart	185	25	10	2	0	B2, B6, B12	Iron, Phosphorus, Zinc	90	75	0.2	0.2
Beef Liver	135	30	5	1	3.8	A, B2, B3, B5, B6, B9, B12, C	Phosphorus, Iron, Zinc, Copper	300	60	0.4	0.3
Beef Loin	275	25	22	9	0	B1, B2, B3, B5, B6, B12	Iron, Zinc, Selenium	100	70	0.1	0.15
Beef Plate	290	22	25	12	0	B1, B2, B3, B5, B6, B12	Iron, Zinc, Selenium	110	75	0.1	0.15

Beef Round	250	26	20	8	0	B1, B2, B3, B5, B6, B12	Iron, Zinc, Selenium	105	70	0.1	0.15
Beef Shank	220	24	16	6	0	B1, B2, B3, B5, B6, B12	Iron, Zinc, Selenium	100	65	0.1	0.15
Beef Tongue	195	20	15	4	0	B1, B2, B3, B5, B6, B12	Iron, Zinc, Selenium	95	60	0.1	0.15
Ground Beef	280	28	22	8	0	B1, B2, B3, B5, B6, B12	Iron, Zinc, Selenium	105	75	0.1	0.15
Ribeye Steak	300	30	25	10	0	B1, B2, B3, B5, B6, B12	Iron, Zinc, Selenium	110	70	0.1	0.15
Ground Pork	290	25	24	10	0	B1, B2, B3, B5, B6, B12	Iron, Zinc, Selenium	95	75	0.2	0.3
Ham	145	17	6	2	1.5	B1, B2, B3, B5, B6, B12	Iron, Zinc, Selenium	70	1100	0.15	0.2
Pork Belly	310	18	28	12	0	B1, B2, B3, B5, B6, B12	Iron, Zinc, Selenium	120	65	0.2	0.3
Pork Chops	260	24	20	9	0	B1, B2, B3, B5, B6, B12	Iron, Zinc, Selenium	90	75	0.2	0.25
Pork Jowl	315	20	30	14	0	B1, B2, B3, B5, B6, B12	Iron, Zinc, Selenium	130	65	0.3	0.35
Pork Liver	165	27	5	1	4	A, B2, B3, B5, B6, B9, B12, C	Phosphorus, Iron, Zinc, Copper	300	60	0.4	0.3
Pork Loin	275	23	24	9	0	B1, B2, B3, B5, B6, B12	Iron, Zinc, Selenium	105	75	0.1	0.15

Pork Ribs	290	22	25	12	0	B1, B2, B3, B5, B6, B12	Iron, Zinc, Selenium	110	75	0.1	0.15
Pork Shoulder	310	21	27	13	0	B1, B2, B3, B5, B6, B12	Iron, Zinc, Selenium	115	75	0.2	0.3
Prosciutto	125	14	7	3	0	B1, B2, B3, B5, B6, B12	Iron, Zinc, Selenium	65	1400	0.2	0.25
Lamb Brains	150	12	10	3	0	B1, B2, B3, B5, B6, B12	Iron, Zinc, Selenium	200	60	0.4	0.3

POULTRY:

Chicken Breast	165	31	3.6	1	0	B3, B6, B12	Phosphorus, Zinc	85	74	0.03	0.7
Chicken Hearts	185	26	8	2.5	0	B2, B6, B12	Iron, Zinc, Copper	170	80	0.1	1
Chicken Legs	175	28	7.9	2.4	0	B3, B6, B12	Phosphorus, Zinc	93	70	0.1	1.5
Chicken Liver	119	16	4.8	1.6	0	A, B2, B3, B6, B12	Iron, Zinc, Copper	345	70	0.1	1.3
Chicken Skin	450	9	40	10	0	B2, B6	Phosphorus, Zinc	100	100	1	8.5
Chicken Thighs	209	26	10.9	3.1	0	B3, B6, B12	Phosphorus, Zinc	109	82	0.1	2.9
Chicken Wings	203	30	16	4.5	0	B3, B6, B12	Phosphorus, Zinc	93	90	0.1	3.7

Duck Breasts	337	20	28	9.7	0	B3, B6, B12	Iron, Zinc	84	60	0.4	3.5
Duck Liver	130	18	5	1.9	0	A, B2, B3, B6, B12	Iron, Zinc, Copper	515	80	0.3	0.7
Ground Turkey	200	23	12	3	0	B3, B6, B12	Phosphorus, Zinc	90	95	0.2	0.9
Turkey Breast	135	30	1	0.3	0	B3, B6, B12	Phosphorus, Zinc	75	70	0.2	0.5

SEAFOOD:

Salmon Roe	240	24.6	14	2.9	4	B12, D, A	Iron, Calcium, Magnesium	588	1500	3.9	0.3
Cod	82	17.8	0.7	0.1	0	B3, B6, B12	Phosphorus, Selenium	43	54	0.2	0.02
Haddock	90	20.7	0.9	0.2	0	B3, B6, B12	Phosphorus, Selenium	65	68	0.2	0.02
Lobster Tails	77	16	0.8	0.2	0	B5, B12	Zinc, Copper	72	296	0.2	0.1
Mackerel	205	19	13.9	3.3	0	B3, B6, D	Iron, Phosphorus	95	90	2.6	0.4
Pollock	111	23	1.2	0.2	0	B3, B6	Phosphorus, Selenium	90	90	0.5	0.1
Salmon	206	22	13	2.5	0	B3, B6, D	Iron, Phosphorus	55	59	1.5	0.4

Sea Bass	97	19	1.5	0.3	0	B3, B6	Phosphorus, Selenium	48	68	0.5	0.1
Shrimp	99	24	0.3	0.1	0	B12, D	Zinc, Iodine	195	111	0.3	0.1
Snapper	100	20	1.3	0.3	0	B3, B6, B12	Phosphorus, Selenium	37	55	0.3	0.1
Squid	92	15.6	1.4	0.4	3.1	B12	Zinc, Copper	233	44	0.4	0.1
Tuna	144	32	4.9	1.3	0	B3, B6, B12	Phosphorus, Selenium	38	50	0.5	0.1

DAIRY & EGGS:

Blue Cheese	353	21	29	19.3	2.3	A, D, B2, B12	Calcium, Phosphorus, Zinc	75	1146	0.25	0.84
Butter	717	0.85	81	51.4	0.06	A, D, E, K	Calcium, Phosphorus	215	11	0.3	2.1
Cheddar Cheese	402	24.9	33.1	21.1	1.3	A, D, B2, B12	Calcium, Phosphorus, Zinc	105	621	0.86	0.94
Cream Cheese	342	6.15	34.4	20.2	4.07	A, B2, B12	Calcium, Phosphorus	110	321	0.1	0.9
Eggs	155	13	11	3.3	1.1	A, B2, B5, B12	Calcium, Phosphorus, Zinc	373	124	0.37	1.2
Gouda Cheese	356	24.9	27.4	17.6	2.2	A, D, B2, B12	Calcium, Phosphorus, Zinc	114	819	0.3	0.93

Gruyère Cheese	413	29	32.3	18.9	0.4	A, D, B2, B12	Calcium, Phosphorus, Zinc	89	119	0.4	0.85
Heavy Cream	340	2.8	36	23	2.7	A, D, K2	Calcium, Phosphorus	130	45	0.1	0.9
Mozzarella Cheese	280	22.2	22.1	13.1	2.2	A, D, B2, B12	Calcium, Phosphorus	89	627	0.37	0.12
Parmesan Cheese	431	38	29	19	4.1	A, D, B2, B12	Calcium, Phosphorus, Zinc	88	1529	0.3	0.95
Sour Cream	198	2.1	19.4	10.1	4.6	A, B2, B12	Calcium, Phosphorus	59	89	0.1	1.2
Swiss Cheese	380	27	28.6	18.1	1.4	A, D, B2, B12	Calcium, Phosphorus, Zinc	89	187	0.35	0.85

FATS & OILS:

Beef Tallow	902	0	100	50	0	A, D, E, K	None	109	0	0.5	2
Duck Fat	900	0	100	33	0	A, D	None	100	0	1	12
Ghee	900	0	100	62	0	A, D, E, K2	None	256	0	1.5	0.5
Pork Fat	902	0	100	39.2	0	A, D, E	None	95	0	0.6	10

MEASUREMENT CONVERSIONS

VOLUME EQUIVALENTS (LIQUID)

US Standard	US Standard (fl oz)	Metric Equivalent (mL, L)
1 teaspoon	0.17 fl oz	5 mL
1 tablespoon	0.50 fl oz	15 mL
cup 1/4	2 fl oz	60 mL
1/3 cup	2.67 fl oz	80 mL
cup 1/2	4 fl oz	120 mL
2/3 cup	5.33 fl oz	160 mL
cup 3/4	6 fl oz	180 mL
1 cup	8 fl oz	240 mL
1 pint (2 cups)	16 fl oz	480 mL
1 quart (4 cups)	32 fl oz	960 mL
1 gallon (16 cups)	128 fl oz	3.8 L

VOLUME EQUIVALENTS (DRY)

US Standard	US Standard (Tbsp, Tsp)	Metric Equivalent (mL)
1/4 teaspoon	0.25 tsp	1.2 mL
1/2 teaspoon	0.5 tsp	2.5 mL
1 teaspoon	1 tsp	5 mL
1 tablespoon	1 tbsp	15 mL
1/8 cup	2 tbsp	30 mL
1/4 cup	4 tbsp	60 mL
1/3 cup	5 tbsp + 1 tsp	80 mL
1/2 cup	8 tbsp	120 mL
2/3 cup	10 tbsp + 2 tsp	160 mL
3/4 cup	12 tbsp	180 mL
1 cup	16 tbsp	240 mL
2 cups (1 pint)	32 tbsp	480 mL
4 cups (1 quart)	64 tbsp	960 mL

OVEN TEMPERATURE

Oven Temperature	Fahrenheit (°F)	Celsius (°C)	Gas Mark
Cool	200°F	90°C	1/4
Very Low	225°F	110°C	1/4
Low	250°F	120°C	1/2
Low	275°F	140°C	1
Moderate	300°F	150°C	2
Moderate	325°F	165°C	3
Moderate	350°F	180°C	4
Moderately Hot	375°F	190°C	5
Hot	400°F	200°C	6
Hot	425°F	220°C	7
Very Hot	450°F	230°C	8
Very Hot	475°F	245°C	9
Extremely Hot	500°F	260°C	10

WEIGHT EQUIVALENTS

Ounces (oz)	Pounds (lb)	Grams (g)	Kilograms (kg)
1 oz	0.0625 lb	28 g	0.028 kg
2 oz	0.125 lb	57 g	0.057 kg
4 oz	0.25 lb	113 g	0.113 kg
8 oz	0.5 lb	227 g	0.227 kg
12 oz	0.75 lb	340 g	0.340 kg
16 oz	1 lb	454 g	0.454 kg
32 oz	2 lb	907 g	0.907 kg
64 oz	4 lb	1814 g	1.814 kg
128 oz	8 lb	3629 g	3.629 kg

RECIPE INDEX

MEATS:

BACON
Bacon-Wrapped Eggs with Soft Cheese, 40
Bacon-Wrapped Filet Mignons, 67
Carnivore Diet Breakfast Tacos, 46
Cheese Balls, 51
Chicken Cordon Bleu Roulade, 90
Duck Roulade with French Herbs, 96
Grilled Lobster Tails with Garlic Butter, 106
Grilled Whole Trout, 105
Pork and Smoked Bacon Casserole with Eggs, 84
Pork Chop with Smoked Bacon Butter, 74
Pork Rind Pancakes, 38

BEEF
Baked Beef Chops with Mayonnaise and Cheese, 72
Beef and Egg Scramble, 35
Beef Bacon-Wrapped Meatloaf, 63
Beef Bone Marrow Custard, 52
Beef Chuck Roast with Rosemary Au Jus, 62
Beef Heart Steaks, 71
Beef Jerky, 59
Beef Omelette, 42
Beef Tenderloin Medallions with Peppercorn Sauce, 70
Boiled Beef Tongue Rolls Stuffed, 115
Coffee-Rubbed Beef Brisket, 64
Grilled Beef Kabobs with Garlic Herb Butter, 61
Grilled Porterhouse Steak, 65
Liver, Tongue, and Eggs Skillet, 116
Meat Assorted Salad with Blue Cheese, 57
Ribeye Steak with Blue Cheese Butter, 69
Smoky Beef Tartare, 66

BEEF BONE MARROW
Beef Bone Marrow Custard, 52
Bone Marrow with Fried Eggs, 39

BEEF BROTH
Beef Chuck Roast with Rosemary Au Jus, 62
Beef Tongue Aspic, 114
Boiled Beef Tongue Rolls Stuffed, 115
Chicken Giblet Gravy, 119
Pork and Smoked Bacon Casserole with Eggs, 84
Stewed Pork in Sour Cream Sauce, 85

BEEF HEART
Beef Heart Steaks, 71
Homemade Tongue, Liver, and Heart Sausages, 120

BEEF LIVER
Homemade Tongue, Liver, and Heart Sausages, 120
Liver Pancakes, 117
Liver, Tongue, and Eggs Skillet, 116

BEEF TONGUE
Beef Tongue Aspic, 114
Boiled Beef Tongue Rolls Stuffed, 115
Homemade Tongue, Liver, and Heart Sausages, 120
Liver, Tongue, and Eggs Skillet, 116

FILET MIGNON
Bacon-Wrapped Filet Mignons, 67
Filet Mignon with Truffle Butter, 68

GROUND BEEF
Beef and Egg Scramble, 35
Beef Omelette, 42
Beef Bacon-Wrapped Meatloaf, 63
Carnivore Breakfast Pizza, 44
Carnivore Diet Breakfast Tacos, 46
Meat Bread, 58

GROUND PORK
Pork Cutlets, 79

HAM
Cheese-Crusted Ham and Egg Sandwich, 45
Chicken Cordon Bleu Roulade, 90

LAMB BRAINS
Lamb Brain Scramble, 118

PORK
Baked Pork Belly, 83
Baked Pork Ribs, 78
Carnivore Pork Skewers, 80
Carnivore Pork Stew, 76
Carnivore Pork Stroganoff Style, 77
Pork and Smoked Bacon Casserole with Eggs, 84
Pork Chop with Smoked Bacon Butter, 74
Pork Curls with Gruyère Cheese, 81
Pork Cutlets, 79
Pork Rind Pancakes, 38
Pork Tenderloin Medallions with Sage Brown Butter, 75

PORK BELLY
Baked Pork Belly, 83
Carnivore Pork Stew, 76

PORK KNUCKLE
Roasted Pork Knuckle, 82

PORK LOIN
Carnivore Pork Skewers, 80
Carnivore Pork Stroganoff Style, 77
Pork Curls with Gruyère Cheese, 81

PORK RINDS
Carnivore Breakfast Pizza, 44
Cheese Balls, 51
Pork Rind Pancakes, 38

PORK SHOULDER
Carnivore Pork Stew, 76
Pork and Smoked Bacon Casserole with Eggs, 84
Stewed Pork in Sour Cream Sauce, 85

PROSCIUTTO
Duck Roulade with French Herbs, 96
Prosciutto-Wrapped Stuffed Turkey, 91

POULTRY:

CHICKEN
Baked Chicken Wings, 87
Chicken Cheese Kebab, 97
Chicken Cordon Bleu Roulade, 90
Chicken Confit, 88
Chicken Fingers, 89
Chicken Fricassee with Creamy Dor Blue Sauce, 98
Chicken Giblet Gravy, 119
Chicken Hearts in Sour Cream, 111
Chicken Liver in Curry Cream Sauce, 112
Chicken Liver Pâté, 113
Chicken Meatballs with Creamy Cheese Sauce, 94
Crispy Baked Fish Sticks, 103
Grilled Lobster Tails with Garlic Butter, 106
Grilled Whole Trout, 105
Meat Assorted Salad with Blue Cheese, 57
Prosciutto-Wrapped Stuffed Turkey, 91
Squid Stuffed, 104

CHICKEN BREAST
Chicken Cordon Bleu Roulade, 90
Chicken Fingers, 89
Chicken Fricassee with Creamy Dor Blue Sauce, 98
Squid Stuffed, 104

CHICKEN GIBLETS
Chicken Giblet Gravy, 119

CHICKEN GIZZARD
Chicken Giblet Gravy, 119

CHICKEN HEARTS
Chicken Hearts in Sour Cream, 111
Chicken Giblet Gravy, 119

CHICKEN LEGS
Chicken Confit, 88

CHICKEN LIVER
Chicken Liver in Curry Cream Sauce, 112
Chicken Liver Pâté, 113
Chicken Giblet Gravy, 119

CHICKEN SKIN
Fried Chicken Skin, 50

CHICKEN WINGS
Baked Chicken Wings, 87

DUCK BREASTS
Duck Roulade with French Herbs, 96

DUCK LIVER
Duck Liver Mousse, 55

GOOSE
Roast Goose with Sage and Thyme, 95

GROUND CHICKEN
Meat Bread, 58
Chicken Cheese Kebab, 97
Chicken Meatballs with Creamy Cheese Sauce, 94

GROUND TURKEY
Meatballs with Cream Sauce, 93

TURKEY BACON
Carnivore Diet Turkey Bacon-Wrapped Mozzarella Sticks, 56

TURKEY BREAST
Prosciutto-Wrapped Stuffed Turkey, 91
Turkey and Cheese Grilled Kebabs, 92

SEAFOOD:

CAVIAR (SALMON ROE)
Salmon Grill with Caviar Sauce, 101

COD
Crispy Baked Fish Sticks, 103

HADDOCK
Crispy Baked Fish Sticks, 103

LOBSTER TAILS
Grilled Lobster Tails with Garlic Butter, 106

MACKEREL
Baked Mackerel and Salmon Rolls, 102

POLLOCK
Crispy Baked Fish Sticks, 103

SALMON
Baked Mackerel and Salmon Rolls, 102
Baked Salmon Slices Wrapped in Bacon, 100
Salmon Grill with Caviar Sauce, 101

SEA BASS
Salt-Baked Fish, 109

SHRIMP
Egg and Shrimp Bake, 37
Squid Stuffed, 104

SNAPPER
Salt-Baked Fish, 109

SQUID
Squid Stuffed, 104

TUNA
Tuna and Egg Salad, 54

DAIRY & EGGS:

BLUE CHEESE
Chicken Fricassee with Creamy Dor Blue Sauce, 98
Meat Assorted Salad with Blue Cheese, 57
Mussels in Blue Cheese Sauce, 108
Ribeye Steak with Blue Cheese Butter, 69

BUTTER
Baked Mussels with Cheese, 107
Beef Tenderloin Medallions with Peppercorn Sauce, 70
Carnivore Pork Stroganoff Style, 77
Chicken Liver Pâté, 113
Creamy Scrambled Eggs, 36
Duck Roulade with French Herbs, 96
Egg and Shrimp Bake, 37
Filet Mignon with Truffle Butter, 68

Grilled Beef Kabobs with Garlic Herb Butter, 61
Grilled Lobster Tails with Garlic Butter, 106
Pork Chop with Smoked Bacon Butter, 74
Pork Rind Pancakes, 38
Pork Tenderloin Medallions with Sage Brown Butter, 75
Ribeye Steak with Blue Cheese Butter, 69

CHEDDAR CHEESE

Baked Beef Chops with Mayonnaise and Cheese, 72
Boiled Beef Tongue Rolls Stuffed, 115
Cheese Balls, 51
Cheese Crispy Roll Stuffed with Soft Cheese, 48
Chicken Cheese Kebab, 97
Chicken Meatballs with Creamy Cheese Sauce, 94
Turkey and Cheese Grilled Kebabs, 92

CREAM CHEESE

Bacon-Wrapped Eggs with Soft Cheese, 40
Cheese Balls, 51
Cheese Crispy Roll Stuffed with Soft Cheese, 48

EGGS

Bacon-Wrapped Eggs with Soft Cheese, 40
Beef and Egg Scramble, 35
Beef Bacon-Wrapped Meatloaf, 63
Beef Bone Marrow Custard, 52
Beef Omelette, 42
Bone Marrow with Fried Eggs, 39
Carnivore Breakfast Pizza, 44
Carnivore Diet Breakfast Tacos, 46
Carnivore Mayonnaise, 53
Cheese-Crusted Ham and Egg Sandwich, 45
Chicken Fingers, 89
Creamy Scrambled Eggs, 36
Crispy Baked Fish Sticks, 103
Deviled Eggs, 49
Egg and Shrimp Bake, 37
Egg Muffins, 41
Homemade Tongue, Liver, and Heart Sausages, 120
Lamb Brain Scramble, 118
Liver Pancakes, 117
Liver Tongue and Eggs Skillet,
Meat Assorted Salad with Blue Cheese, 57
Meat Bread, 58
Pork and Smoked Bacon Casserole with Eggs, 84
Pork Cutlets, 79
Pork Rind Pancakes, 38
Salt-Baked Fish, 109
Sausage Scramble, 43
Smoky Beef Tartare, 66
Tuna and Egg Salad, 54

GOUDA CHEESE

Cheese Balls, 51

GRUYÈRE CHEESE

Baked Mussels with Cheese, 107
Pork Curls with Gruyère Cheese, 81

HEAVY CREAM

Baked Mussels with Cheese, 107
Beef Bone Marrow Custard, 52
Beef Tenderloin Medallions with Peppercorn Sauce, 70
Carnivore Pork Stroganoff Style, 77
Chicken Fricassee with Creamy Dor Blue Sauce, 98
Chicken Liver in Curry Cream Sauce, 112
Chicken Liver Pâté, 113
Chicken Meatballs with Creamy Cheese Sauce, 94
Creamy Scrambled Eggs, 36
Pork Rind Pancakes, 38
Meatballs with Cream Sauce, 93
Salmon Grill with Caviar Sauce, 101
Smoky Beef Tartare, 66

MOZZARELLA CHEESE

Baked Beef Chops with Mayonnaise and Cheese, 72
Boiled Beef Tongue Rolls Stuffed, 115
Carnivore Diet Turkey Bacon-Wrapped Mozzarella Sticks, 56
Cheese Balls, 51
Chicken Cheese Kebab, 97
Chicken Meatballs with Creamy Cheese Sauce, 94
Prosciutto-Wrapped Stuffed Turkey, 91
Turkey and Cheese Grilled Kebabs, 92

PARMESAN CHEESE

Baked Mussels with Cheese, 107

Cheese Crispy Roll Stuffed with Soft Cheese, 48
Chicken Fingers, 89
Crispy Baked Fish Sticks, 103

SOUR CREAM

Chicken Hearts in Sour Cream, 111
Stewed Pork in Sour Cream Sauce, 85

SWISS CHEESE

Chicken Cordon Bleu Roulade, 90

FATS & OILS:

BACON FAT

Chicken Cordon Bleu Roulade, 90
Smoky Beef Tartare, 66
Squid Stuffed, 104
Grilled Whole Trout, 105

BEEF TALLOW

Baked Chicken Wings, 87
Baked Mackerel and Salmon Rolls, 102
Baked Mussels with Cheese, 107
Baked Pork Belly, 83
Beef and Egg Scramble, 35
Beef Bone Marrow Custard, 52
Beef Heart Steaks, 71
Beef Omelette, 42
Beef Tenderloin Medallions with Peppercorn Sauce, 70
Bone Marrow with Fried Eggs, 39
Carnivore Breakfast Pizza, 44
Carnivore Diet Breakfast Tacos, 46
Chicken Cheese Kebab, 97
Chicken Fricassee with Creamy Dor Blue Sauce, 98
Chicken Giblet Gravy, 119
Chicken Liver in Curry Cream Sauce, 112
Chicken Liver Pâté, 113
Creamy Scrambled Eggs, 36
Egg Muffins, 41
Fried Chicken Skin, 50
Grilled Porterhouse Steak, 65
Lamb Brain Scramble, 118
Liver, Tongue, and Eggs Skillet, 116
Meatballs with Cream Sauce, 93

Pork and Smoked Bacon Casserole with Eggs, 84
Pork Cutlets, 79
Pork Rind Pancakes, 38
Salt-Baked Fish, 109
Salmon Grill with Caviar Sauce, 101
Smoky Beef Tartare, 66

CHICKEN FAT

Chicken Confit, 88

DUCK FAT

Chicken Confit, 88
Duck Liver Mousse, 55
Duck Roulade with French Herbs, 96

GHEE

Beef Tenderloin Medallions with Peppercorn Sauce, 70
Chicken Giblet Gravy, 119
Chicken Hearts in Sour Cream, 111
Chicken Liver in Curry Cream Sauce, 112
Grilled Whole Trout, 105
Homemade Tongue, Liver, and Heart Sausages, 120
Lamb Brain Scramble, 118
Liver Pancakes, 117
Liver, Tongue, and Eggs Skillet, 116
Squid Stuffed, 104

MAYONNAISE

Baked Beef Chops with Mayonnaise and Cheese, 72
Boiled Beef Tongue Rolls Stuffed, 115
Deviled Eggs, 49
Meat Assorted Salad with Blue Cheese, 57
Tuna and Egg Salad, 54

PORK LARD

Baked Chicken Wings, 87
Baked Mackerel and Salmon Rolls, 102
Carnivore Pork Skewers, 80
Chicken Cheese Kebab, 97
Chicken Cordon Bleu Roulade, 90
Chicken Fricassee with Creamy Dor Blue Sauce, 98
Chicken Meatballs with Creamy Cheese Sauce, 94
Meatballs with Cream Sauce, 93

Pork and Smoked Bacon Casserole with Eggs, 84
Pork Cutlets, 79
Prosciutto-Wrapped Stuffed Turkey, 91
Salmon Grill with Caviar Sauce, 101
Stewed Pork in Sour Cream Sauce, 85

SPICES & SEASONINGS:

BLACK PEPPER
All the Dishes or to Taste

COFFEE GROUNDS
Coffee-Rubbed Beef Brisket, 64

CURRY POWDER
Chicken Liver in Curry Cream Sauce, 112

DILL
Baked Mackerel and Salmon Rolls, 102
Salt-Baked Fish, 109

GARLIC
Chicken Confit, 88
Grilled Beef Kabobs with Garlic Herb Butter, 61
Grilled Lobster Tails with Garlic Butter, 106
Roast Goose with Sage and Thyme, 95

GARLIC POWDER
Beef Jerky, 59
Chicken Fingers, 89
Carnivore Pork Stew, 76

LEMON JUICE
Carnivore Mayonnaise, 53
Grilled Lobster Tails with Garlic Butter, 106

MUSTARD POWDER
Smoky Beef Tartare, 66

ONION POWDER
Beef Jerky, 59

PAPRIKA
Chicken Fingers, 89
Smoky Beef Tartare, 66

PARSLEY
Baked Mackerel and Salmon Rolls, 102
Duck Roulade with French Herbs, 96
Grilled Beef Kabobs with Garlic Herb Butter, 61
Mussels in Blue Cheese Sauce, 108

PEPPERCORNS
Beef Tenderloin Medallions with Peppercorn Sauce, 70

ROSEMARY
Beef Chuck Roast with Rosemary Au Jus, 62
Duck Roulade with French Herbs, 96
Grilled Beef Kabobs with Garlic Herb Butter, 61
Roast Goose with Sage and Thyme, 95
Salt-Baked Fish, 109

SALT
All the Dishes or to Taste

THYME
Chicken Confit, 88
Duck Roulade with French Herbs, 96
Grilled Beef Kabobs with Garlic Herb Butter, 61
Roast Goose with Sage and Thyme, 95
Salt-Baked Fish, 109
Carnivore Pork Stew, 76

LEAVE A REVIEW – YOUR VOICE MATTERS!

Thank you for joining me on this flavorful journey through **The Carnivore Instinct. Cookbook for Beginners!** I hope you've enjoyed exploring the world of meat-based nutrition and that the recipes have made your carnivore lifestyle easier and more delicious.

If this book has helped you, I'd love to hear your thoughts. Whether you've tried just one recipe or embraced a whole new way of eating, your feedback means the world to me and will help others, too.

WHY LEAVE A REVIEW?

- **Share Your Experience** – Let others know how this book has impacted your health and cooking habits.
- **Help Others** – Your review can guide fellow carnivores or those curious about the diet to make informed decisions.
- **Support Me** – Honest feedback allows me to improve future editions and continue creating valuable content for people like you.

WHERE TO LEAVE YOUR REVIEW:

- Head over to Amazon.com or your favorite online retailer where you purchased the book.
- Share your thoughts on social media and tag me @CarnivoreInstinct!

Your review means so much, and I appreciate you taking the time to help spread the word about living a simpler, healthier, and meat-filled life.

Thank you for being a part of this carnivore journey with me!

With gratitude,
Garrett Lane

LEAVE A REVIEW ON AMAZON:

United States	Canada	United Kingdom	Australia

Printed in Great Britain
by Amazon